Story Re-Visions

STORY RE-VISIONS

*Narrative Therapy in
the Postmodern World*

ALAN PARRY
ROBERT E. DOAN

THE GUILFORD PRESS
New York   London

Printed in the United States of America

This book is printed on acid-free paper.

Last digit is print number: 9 8 7 6 5 4 3 2

Library of Congress Cataloging-in-Publication Data

Parry, Alan (Thomas Alan)
    Story re-visions: narrative therapy in the postmodern world /
Alan Parry, Robert E. Doan.
        p.   cm.
    Includes bibliographical references and index.
    ISBN 0-89862-213-1.—ISBN 0-89862-570-X (pbk.)
    1. Storytelling—Therapeutic use. 2. Postmodernism—Psychological
aspects. 3. Personal construct therapy. 4. Family psychotherapy.
I. Doan, Robert E. II. Title.
RC489.S74P37 1994
616.89′14′01—dc20   94-18296
                                                        CIP

Preface

This book began as a series of conversations about narrative therapy between two friends who get to see each other only once or twice a year due to the geographical distance between their residences. On such occasions, it was discovered that most of Alan Parry's discussion centered upon the philosophical and literary basis of narrative, while Rob Doan talked mostly about translating narrative ideas into the actual practice of therapy. This led to Alan suggesting that a merging of such conversations might make for a very useful book. That idea took root. The outcome is really two books in one, each written in the language and style of the respective authors. The book, therefore, contains two distinct voices which, in spite of deep friendship and philosophical brotherhood, find quite different modes of expression in the domains of the language and performance of therapy. This seems entirely in keeping with the intention of writing a postmodern reflection on narrative therapy.

The book begins in the voice of Alan Parry chanting the postmodern into being, tracing its evolution across time and disciplines. It continues with him setting the stage for the challenge of doing therapy in a world that modernity has largely destoried, leaving us unsettled postmoderns to re-story in personal and local ways. Rob Doan then takes up the chant, introducing a change of voice and rhythm which offers specific guidelines for the "re-vision" of personal stories for both clients and therapists. Though the voices are different, they are attuned to the same melody. It is hoped the reader will experience their joining as harmonious.

At the completion of any book, some acknowledgments are in order. Alan Parry is indebted to his father for having been such a wonderful storyteller and to his mother for passing on her fascination with people and their stories. He would also like to thank Dr. Roy Fairchild, his teacher during his doctoral studies and mentor in the years since, for giving him confidence in his own ideas. He thanks Elke, his partner, muse, and first editor, whose insistent belief in him made his contribution to this book possible; and their children—Shannon, Peter, David, Robert, Richard, Sybil, and Karen—their partners, and two grandchildren—Benjamin and Sophie—all of whom demonstrate daily the magic that can arise when stories are connected from different families and diverse traditions.

Alan would also like to thank Myrna Fraser and Beverly Anderson for their patience and good humor in helping him develop his otherwise primitive computer skills so that he could write with dispatch and enjoyment. He would like to express his appreciation to Karl Tomm for creating a context of rare intellectual excitement and neverending curiosity, which has provided a fertile ground for the growth of new ideas and practices.

Rob Doan would like to thank his parents for providing him with a world that made pursuing a higher education possible, and the myriad of teachers who have informed his thinking over the years. He would also like to thank Monte, who has been not only an understanding partner in the writing of this book, but also an equal and able partner in the wild, postmodern ride they have taken together over the years. And last, but not least, thanks to Lorin for her love.

Finally, Alan and Rob would like to thank Seymour Weingarten, Editor-in-Chief of The Guilford Press, for his original initiative and continuing interest on behalf of this book, and Judith Grauman for overseeing the final stages of production. They also appreciate the assiduous and helpful copy editing by Marie Sprayberry, who did a beautiful job of ironing out tangled passages and helped make the final outcome a book that Alan and Rob are both proud of. Thanks to her, the authors are able to rest much more confident in the hope that reading *Story Re-Visions* will be a stimulating and profitable experience.

ALAN PARRY
ROBERT E. DOAN

Contents

1. The Postmodern Context   1

   The Narrative and the Paradigmatic Traditions, 1
   Modernism and the Quest for Inner Truth, 6
   A Delegitimized World, 9

2. Doing Narrative Therapy in a Destoried World   12

   Many Worlds, Many Selves: Toward Postmodernism
   in Family Therapy, 12
   A Therapy Equal to Postmodern Challenges, 22
   What Narrative Can Still Do, 26
   Postmodern Ethics and the Mystery of the Other, 30
   Old Stories and Their Re-Vision, 33

3. Helping People Become Authors of Their Own Stories   44

   The Importance of Story Re-Vision, 45
   Our Definition of Family Therapy, 47
   Case Background, 48
   Tools for Inviting Clients to Become Authors, 49
   Concluding Comment, 84
   Appendix: Therapeutic Examples, 84

4. The Therapist and Reflecting Team as Re-Visionary Editors   118

   The Therapist as Re-Visionary Editor, 119
   Guidelines for the Re-Visionary Therapist/Editor, 121
   The Reflecting Team as an Editorial Committee, 130
   Appendix: Therapeutic Examples, 136

5. Keeping the Story Re-Vision Alive, Well, and in Charge   157

   Recruiting an Audience for the New Story, 158
   Using Letters to Consolidate New Story Roles, 167
   Staying Behind the Client, 168

Re-Visioning Clients as Experts on Their Own Stories, 170
Concluding Comment, 173
Appendix: Therapeutic Examples, 173

6. The Re-Vision of Therapists' Stories in Training
and Supervision   187
The Re-Vision of Therapists' Stories about Clients, 189
The Re-Vision of Therapists' Stories about Themselves, 191
Helping Other Therapists Re-Vision Their Stories, 192
Concluding Comment, 194
Appendix: Therapeutic Examples, 195

References   206

Index   212

CHAPTER 1

The Postmodern Context

Those like Slothrop, with the greatest interest in discovering the truth, were thrown back on dreams, psychic flashes, omens, cryptographies, drug-epistemologies, all dancing on a ground of terror, contradiction, and absurdity.
—THOMAS PYNCHON, *Gravity's Rainbow* (1973, p. 583)

THE NARRATIVE
AND THE PARADIGMATIC TRADITIONS

Once upon a time, everything was understood through stories. Stories were always called upon to make things understandable. The philosopher Friedrich Nietzsche once said that "if we possess our *why* of life we can put up with almost any *how*" (1889/1968, p. 23). Stories always dealt with the "why" questions. The answers they gave did not have to be literally true; they only had to satisfy people's curiosity by providing an answer, less for the mind than for the soul. For the soul they were true, but probably no one bothered to ask whether that truth was factual or "merely" metaphorical. That question came much later.

Most of the first questions were about origins: "Why is there something and not nothing?" "How did we get here?" "Who made the world, and why?" "Why did we get divided up into males and females?" "Why did trouble and sorrow enter the world?" "Why do we have to work instead of just enjoying the world's plenty?" "Why do women have pain in childbirth yet animals do not?" Before the modern era, all peoples of the world, whatever their level of sophistication or lack of it, attempted to answer these and other "big questions" through stories. People raised within the Western, Judeo-Christian tradition have generally been most familiar with the stories contained within the first three chapters of *Genesis*, the first book of the Bible. The Biblical stories of the origin of things and of our follies and failings give, virtually without exception, a distinctly *moral* dimension to the answers they provide. Folly and pain come to humankind, for instance, not through blind fate or some capricious impulse of God, but because Adam and Eve cannot observe even the one limitation placed upon them by the Creator. The creation stories of other peoples, by contrast, sometimes appear to have a whimsical quality to them: In the Haida story of the origins of humanity, for instance, Raven displays a knockabout curiosity in picking with his beak at a particularly lively and potentially delicious clam, within which is contained not a meal, but the first people.

All such stories have in common, however serious or whimsical, a quality of sufficiency. They give an answer to one of the big "why" questions in a way that most fully accounts for the implications of the question through images that make life meaningful within that culture. In other words, it is the *meaningfulness* of the answers given, rather than their factual *truthfulness*, that gives them their credibility. The hearers of the story believed that it was true because it was meaningful, rather that it was meaningful because it was true.

The pursuit of truth over meaning as humankind's highest achievement probably began with Plato. This represents the introduction into the world of what the psychologist Jerome Bruner (1986) has described as the "paradigmatic" as opposed to the "narrative" mode of cognition. Bruner identifies these as nothing less than "two modes of cognitive functioning, two modes of thought. Each provide distinct ways of ordering experience, of constructing reality. The two (though complementary) are irreducible to one another" (p. 11). He goes on to define the paradigmatic or logico-scientific mode acccording to its "attempts to fulfill the ideal of a formal, mathematical system of description and explanation. It employs categorization or conceptualization and the operations by which categories are established, instantiated, idealized and related one to the other to form a system" (p. 12). Its aim is the establishment of truth, whereas the narrative mode seeks to convince on the basis of what he calls "verisimilitude" or "lifelikeness." Narrative also convinces, we ourselves would add, because it provides a web of meaning and of connectedness to events, which reassures people that things happen as they do because they take place in a moral universe. As such, the narrative mode deals with what Bruner refers to as "the vicissitudes of intention" (p. 17). In our view, this is the proper domain of therapy: how people feel about themselves when their actions repeatedly fail to match their intentions, or their intentions fail to measure up to their aspirations. It follows that narratives are conversations about the dramatic ironies to which intentions are susceptible—the many ways in which they surprise and confound people. As such, the subject matter of therapeutic conversation is, invariably, intentions gone awry.

Alasdair MacIntyre (1981) suggests that "conversation, understood widely enough, is the form of human transactions in general." To this he adds, "I am presenting both conversations in particular then and human actions in general as *enacted narratives*" (p. 211; emphasis added). He quotes Barbara Hardy, who says that "we dream in narrative, day-dream in narrative, remember, anticipate, hope, despair, believe, doubt, plan, revise, criticize, construct, gossip, learn, hate and love by narrative" (MacIntyre, 1981, p. 211). Finally, MacIntyre too relates narrative to intentionality when he says that "behavior is only characterized adequately when we know what the longer- and longest-term intentions invoked are and how the shorter-term intentions are related to the longer. Once again we are involved in writing a narrative history" (p. 208).

The eminent hermeneuticist Paul Ricoeur, in the first volume of his three-volume work *Time and Narrative* (1984), suggest that narrative is inescapably linked to the temporal domain, such that "time becomes human time to the extent that it is organized after the manner of a narrative" (p. 3). Elsewhere he suggests that "to compose a story is, from the temporal point of view, to derive a configuration from a succession" (1987/1991a, p. 427). It is to give a life intelligibility by placing it on a meaningful continuum containing a past, a present, and a future, which are linked by a particular quality. We agree with Bruner and with MacIntyre in identifying this quality as intentionality, which makes it possible for people to plot the course of their lives according to their own choices, rather than in reaction to the initiatives of others. The latter is what occurs when people respond before checking in with their own intentions, which alone allow them to enact their own narratives instead of serving only as characters in other people's narratives. Even the most goal-directed individuals, however, must deal with the contingencies that require them to improvise, change direction, and reformulate meanings. Such changes, even when unwelcome, contribute to a richer, deeper, more interesting, better-plotted narrative. What could be more deadly, after all, than a life in which outcomes always match intentions? A rich, varied, and polysemic use of language is a profound asset in the living of a well-plotted narrative. Ricoeur suggests the word "poetry" for such language, "in the sense that the plot of a narrative is a creation of productive imagination which projects a world of its own. And the stories are no less poetry than versified literature" (1982/1991b, p. 452).

The paradigmatic mode of cognition makes a poor language for describing human action and interaction. It is, to be sure, indispensable for what Gregory Bateson (1972) calls the world of the "nonliving," in contrast to the world of the "living." Ricoeur calls paradigmatic language the language of instrumentalization and describes it as the most dangerous trend of our culture. We have only one model of language—the language of science and technology (1982/1991b, p. 448). Scientific language seeks, of necessity, to reduce a word to a single meaning. "But," Ricoeur goes on, "it is the task of poetry [or narrative] to make words mean as much as they can and not as little as they can. Therefore, [the aim is] not to elude or exclude this plurivocity, but to cultivate it, to make it meaningful, powerful, and therefore to bring back to language all its capacity of meaningfulness" (1982/1991b, p. 449). Yet psychotherapy, in its efforts to legitimize itself as truly scientific and hence "truthful," still tends to theorize scientifically for an activity that is inescapably narrative in its subject matter, thereby establishing the foundations of its practice exclusively in paradigmatic language. Such foundationalism is one of the hallmarks of Western thought, and at the same time one of the chief casualties of the postmodern temper. J.-F. Lyotard (1984) makes the claim, however, that it has traditionally taken what he calls a "grand narrative" or "metanarrative" to legitimize paradigmatic systems in philosophy and later science.

We do not deride paradigmatic thinking. Quite apart from the wonders it has made possible through the discoveries of science and the inventions of technology, the critical thinking made possible by its precision and exactitude has itself contributed to the liberation of narrative. Sacred stories in particular take on a sacrosanct quality, which leads to the subordination of their meaningfulness to their unquestioned truthfulness. The inexorable forward movement of modernity, with its virtual idolization of the paradigmatic mode, made it all but inevitable that eventually even the Bible, the dominant sacred narrative of the West, would be subjected to its critical methods. In fact, all of the grand narratives that have variously inspired Western civilization have been thrown into question in regard to their claims of truth. Although this has opened a great vacuum of meaning at the heart of this civilization, it has also succeeded in liberating many of these stories—indeed, the very way stories can be told—from the tyranny of having to be legitimized by a metanarrative before they can be taken seriously. The celebration of this freedom is abundantly evident in the best works of postmodern fiction, such as *One Hundred Years of Solitude* by Gabriel Garcia Marquez (1970), *Gravity's Rainbow* by Thomas Pynchon (1973), and *Midnight's Children* by Salman Rushdie (1981).

Something similar is happening in family therapy, which, in our view, is for postmodernism what psychoanalysis was for modernism. Michael White's (1986) introduction of the practice of externalizing the problem has the effect of personifying the constraint that is binding the family. Thus, when a particular child is described as being under the influence of "trouble," so that its various tricks send a "reputation" ahead of the child, it begins to take on the qualities of a treacherous person who has taken hold in the family, rather than those of a clinical symptom. In a recent article entitled " 'If You Were a Problem,' " Christopher Kinman (1994) has taken the appropriate step and built a significant intervention around the characterization of the problem as, in effect, "the man who came to dinner" and now has the whole family tied in knots of anger and recrimination. Similarly, Tomm (1990) suggests that instead of viewing families and other significant groups as collections of separate individuals, we should begin to view individuals as communities of "internalized others," in a manner reminiscent of Norman O. Brown's Dionysian *Love's Body* (1966): "Every person, then, is many persons; a multitude made into one person; a corporate body; incorporated, a corporation" (Brown, 1966, p. 147). Kinman (1993) asks troubled adolescents to tell their stories not from their own point of view, but from those of several internalized others (such as parents, friends, and probation officers). Our own work abounds with challenges to the single, dominant story by inviting our clients to imagine many other stories drawn from the texts of the lives of those with whom the clients are in intense interaction. When the very notion that there is one true story is thrown into question, people begin to realize that any story is just a story. They are freed to invent stories of their own that serve the purpose of any narrative: to provide a framework of meaning and direction so that a life may be lived intentionally.

This was not always so, of course. Stories that were once liberating often became tyrannizing, especially to the extent that they claimed to be *the* one true story. This was (and often still is) a pursuit that the Western world seems to have found particularly congenial, stemming from two streams—one philosophical, the other religious—determined upon the single-minded quest for that one truth. Yet as long as the Christian story was dominant in the Western world, people were able to live their lives intentionally by experiencing themselves as characters within that story and interpreting events in their lives in terms of the meaning provided by Christianity's dramatic and cosmic events. Thus, however mean or modest people might be, they believed themselves to be participants in a cosmic drama, persons whose actions and even whose thoughts were of concern to the Creator of the universe Himself. What could have been more consoling and meaningful than that? It would never have occurred to people living within this sacred story (or any other one, for that matter) that life could ever be free of sorrow or tragedy, much less of frustration or frequent privation. Life was by no means expected to be comfortable, and desires were not expected to be met as a matter of course. Trials were expected, not only to test but to strengthen a pilgrim's soul, and were almost welcomed.

MODERNISM AND THE QUEST
FOR INNER TRUTH

Modernity challenged the sacred story at almost every point. It was a time of breathtaking change such as the world had never known or even imagined. In a sense, it was a celebration of transience and impermanence. But, given the historic Western preoccupation with *the* one true story, it must have seemed quite impossible to let the situation be. A foundation of sameness, certainty, and truth and a correspondence between the inner and the outer had to be found, so that the inner person who was being so neglected by the external gaze of modernity could find a familiar place upon which to stand amidst the uncertainties created by the repeated challenges (explicit and implicit) to the Christian story, which had for so long provided that foundation of certainty for the soul. The answer of the modernist artists, who began to emerge at the very apex of the Western world's strident confidence in itself, was to suggest a new approach to old certainties, while at the same time challenging every complacent certainty that the proud world of the triumphant Western bourgeoisie was resting upon.

The work of these artists offered a compass for the inner person, to enable him/her[1] to move with the external forces of irresistible change that were sweeping the world. In so doing, however, they (probably unintentionally) set modernity on its final form of expression: the release of the individual from every kind of social, religious, political, and economic restraint that had characterized the medieval world. All that was now left was the naked self of a human being who, by virtue of the miracles wrought by science and technology on the one hand, and religious and political freedom on the other, was free to live almost exclusively for personal freedom and gratification.

Into this void came Sigmund Freud, who, in the words of the poet W. H. Auden, became "no more a person now, but a whole climate of opinion" (1939/1966, p. 168). To begin with, Freud spoke as aptly as he did for the times by attempting to straddle the world of science and that of literary art, and succeeded in this endeavor for the most part. It must be acknowledged, however, that he wears better today as an artist and philosopher than as a scientist. Be that as it may, Freud's interest for the narrative therapist is that he began simply to listen to the stories told by people who found themselves carrying around and using other people's words—primarily those of their parents, as well as the strictures of society—to describe their own experiences. Moreover, for these individuals' parents, words were unduly constraining and meaningless amidst the changes

---

[1]We prefer to honor the value of gender neutrally by alternating from one passage to the next between placing masculine pronouns first ("him/her") and feminine pronouns first ("her/him") in reference to a generic human being. We do this through the remainder of the text.

of modernity. When Freud let the words flow freely, in ways strikingly similar to those found in the fiction of James Joyce and Marcel Proust, people would stumble over suddenly unaccountable gaps in their stories. If he then either waited patiently or prodded gently and without moral judgment, those gaps would be filled by forgotten experiences, which often were at shocking variance with the versions that had been put in the individuals' mouths by others. Suddenly their own versions of lost experiences enabled them to find their own voices to describe their own experiences. Their lives began to make sense, and they had stories of their own; they were no longer compelled to live as supporting characters in stories that had gone forward at their expense. In this sense, too, Freud was a modernist, adhering to the faith that if his patients probed deeply enough they would *find* the answers they were looking for: in the unconscious. Moreover, he believed that once these forsaken stories stored in the unconscious were restored to consciousness, the interferences and their resulting distortions that they had created in the individuals' understanding of the world could end, and their perceptions would once again correspond to reality as it was.

As such, Freud must be counted as the first narrative therapist. This has already been implicitly admitted by the acknowledgment of his creation of a new literary genre, the case history; by his being accorded the honor he most cherished, the Goethe Prize for literary merit; and by the fact that he was nominated for a Nobel Prize in literature rather than medicine. But he was equally determined to be a scientist. He persisted in formulating his discoveries in paradigmatic language, and, wholly unlike an artist, he insisted on the *truth* (albeit evolving) of his theories. Like any modernist, he insisted furthermore on providing a paradigmatic foundation for the dynamism of the stories he heard from his patients. Of course, wherever there is an underlying foundational theory of truth, there must be an expert to interpret it. When the area of supposed expertise is another person's experiences, the expert is, ironically, taking that persons voice away from her/him. Thus, what Freud gave away with one hand he took back with the other, and virtually the entire succeeding field of psychotherapy followed him. The therapist became the expert on each client—the one a person went to when the emptied self of modernity's pace became unbearably anxious because it no longer belonged to any meaning-lending story and had no story of its own.

A DELEGITIMIZED WORLD

The modernist gospel of the liberated self and the necessity of its own esteem remains perhaps one of the few widespread metanarratives that is still alive and more or less well. The same cannot be said for some of the grand secular stories that developed in the wake of the waning hold of the dominant sacred story. The credibility of a narrative that could have been entitled "Science as the Hope of a Better Future" was challenged by Hiroshima and the threat of nuclear holocaust that haunted the world for the next 45 years. A story of "Progress" has been shattered by the course of world and social events since the end of the 1960s—probably the last period during which it was still believed that the trajectory of history would take us almost inevitably to a better world. Likewise, a story of "Democracy and the Triumph of the People" has been rudely shaken, at least in the Western world, by the growing disillusionment with politicians. People seem to have forgotten in this ahistorical age that politics is merely the "art of the possible." This is perhaps understandable at a time in which desire is king and media capitalism (Jameson, 1991) is able to convince people that what they want is what the impersonal network of power relations referred to by Thomas Pynchon (1973) as "Them" wants them to want. The only stories that remain to give meaning to our lives and legitimacy to our obligations are our own personal stories. The free expression of these stories is legitimized—rather feebly, to be sure—by the "little narrative" (as Lyotard and others might call it) that could perhaps be entitled "The Self and Its Esteem."

We currently find ourselves, therefore, trying to find our bearings in an unprecedented situation: a world without legitimacy. By this we mean that no person, group, or institution, whether political, economic, religious, or sociocultural, commands either trust or credibility sufficient to elicit the voluntary response of a societal consensus. Indeed, suspicion and skepticism toward any individual or group making grand claims seem to be the order of the day. Thus, local points of view, which often seem conspiratorial or victimized in tone, flourish in the postmodern climate precisely *because* those who share such stories experience themselves as lacking in power. Their stories are invented to try to account for this lack, which itself seems one of the prime characteristics accompanying postmodernity:

a sense that *someone* must be in charge. That "someone" is usually all those who are benefiting, and are therefore probably even in control; as such, they are thought to be wielding power *illegitimately.* "Conspiracy," says Fredric Jameson, "is the poor person's cognitive mapping in the postmodern age" (quoted in McHale, 1992, p. 178). The prevalence of conspiratorial themes in postmodern fiction draws upon this mood, which runs through the writings of Thomas Pynchon, William S. Burroughs, Don DeLillo, and John Barth; the popular fiction of Tom Clancy and Robert Ludlum; and the "cyberpunk" science fiction of William Gibson, Bruce Sterling, and many others. It is also found in the wake of one of the most heartening developments of the postmodern era: the demarginalization of those peoples and groups traditionally relegated to the compromised status of "the Other." Many such individuals account for their historic predicament as well as for their present struggles by positing a conspiracy of heterosexual European males. A sense of victimhood abounds. This indicates that people do not perceive themselves as part of their own narratives; instead, they feel excluded from any role except that of scapegoat in the traditional narratives. They feel like characters in other people's stories.

Thus, the loss in authority of the grand narratives may be another of those forces that, by liberating such stories from their historic role as legitimizers of entrenched moral and economic power, makes them available to challenge those whose power seems of questionable legitimacy. Thus the Christian story, for instance, which stood for 1,500 years as the central legitimizing narrative for those holding ecclesiastical, political, and even economic power, has been increasingly freed to give voice to those who are derelict and oppressed—precisely the ones to whom the story was once addressed as good news.

A delegitimized, postmodern world is a place without any single claim to a truth universally respected, and a growing realization that no single story sums up the meaning of life. It is also a place in which so much is happening to so many so fast that no story or theory is sufficient to correspond fully to its subject matter. In some ways, the latter realization is an even greater shock to our ways of understanding than is the loss of a sense of a single truth. If Western thought since Plato has been obsessive in its quest for that single truth, it has been equally bent upon establishing that a full correspondence exists between our view of the world and the world itself. Coming at the theme of correspondence from opposite poles—one defending and one scorning the oppressed, and thereby damning and praising the strong and the ruthless, respectively—Marx and Nietzsche exposed the role that interest and desire play in how we perceive the world. Each from his own perspective asked the shattering question: "*Whose* truth?" Moreover, the implications of Einstein's theory of relativity and Heisenberg's uncertainty principle (although these theories were applied to the macro- and microuniverses, respectively) cast doubt in the name of science itself on the very possibility of objectivity under even the most detached and disinterested of circumstances. Finally, the modern grand narratives of science, progress, and democracy were shown—in spite of their magnificent contributions to a better and more just life for so many—to fall short of their promises. In other words, not only were these stories unable any longer to provide a sense of legitimacy; they were no longer capable of corresponding to the sheer complexity of the very world they had once been able to legitimize and explain. With this, modernism becomes intelligible as the last attempt to preserve the sacred and mythic narratives of the Western tradition. The modernists sought to do this by psychologizing these stories in order to preserve their legitimizing and explanatory power. The inexorable force of modernity itself once again overrode this intention, by giving rise to a world that moved so fast that even these psychologized and deliteralized versions of the old stories could no longer keep up. This has left us in a world in which no single story, however understood, is able to provide either legitimacy or sufficiency equal to the pace of change through what Fredric Jameson (1991) refer to as "hyperspace." The challenges of doing therapy in hyperspace constitute the topic of the next chapter.

CHAPTER 2

Doing Narrative Therapy in a Destoried World

MANY WORLDS, MANY SELVES: TOWARD POSTMODERNISM IN FAMILY THERAPY

Modernist Assumptions and Therapeutic Aims

Traveling through hyperspace—an apt metaphor for trying to keep up with modernity's ever-accelerating pace—can be exceedingly disorienting and frightening. It is particularly challenging for us as therapists. In the first place, it challenges many of our own most basic operating asssumptions. The most fundamental of these are the following: that there is one self per person; that this self is knowable and can be understood and even mastered by the person if only he/she and a therapist go at it long enough; and that people can understand one another with reasonable accuracy. The final assumption would seem to be that people all basically inhabit the same world and that if they can just talk to one another, using the same more or less common language, they can resolve conflicts and misunderstandings and live together in imperfect but acceptable harmony. At the root of these are the modernist assumptions of psychoanalysis, which are, despite the revolutionary agenda of modernism, merely the most recent developments of the tradition that goes back to Plato: that there is a truth of things that can be reached by human thought, which is capable of grasping the essentials of the world that it thinks about. In a word, this tradition is that human thought is capable of establishing a correspondence between itself and the world it observes.

Apparently, Freud and his successors, by accident more than design, used the propensity of human beings to describe themselves narratively as the means by which people could come to know themselves, and, in knowing themselves, know the world better. Freud scorned the term "self" as too nebulous, although he freely used the German word *Seele;* this translates best into English as "soul," but was rendered instead as "mind" in the authorized translations. For Freud, the object of the quest was the unconscious—a term whose mystique could never be denied, however scientific he and his followers insisted it was. It was C. G. Jung who first introduced the term "self" as signifying the central human motivating force. Otto Rank—the most undeservedly overlooked of Freud's rebellious "sons," who in turn influenced Carl Rogers—developed its use further until the self took over, in one way or another, all non- and neo-Freudian psychotherapies. To the extent, then, that therapists of any school continue to operate within assumptions of single selfhood and its essential knowability, they remain steadfastly within a modernist sensibility. This is neither criminal nor heretical, but neither is the distinction between modernist and postmodernist arbitrary. It has tangible implications for the daily work of therapists, particularly if they work with families who live in many worlds and must call upon not one self, but their many selves to navigate across these many worlds.

Postmodernity seems to have been described most aptly thus far by those who are responding more whimsically to the destabilized conditions to which this term has been applied—those who can still smile in the face of the apocalyptic imagery that abounds throughout its literature and art. One of these is a poet, composer, performance artist, and small-press publisher named Dick Higgins, who uses the rubric "cognitive" and "postcognitive" to draw a distinction between modernist and postmodernist. Brian McHale, in an admiring discussion of Higgins, suggests instead the terms "epistemological" and "ontological" to construct the division between the two "eras." Readers who look at Higgins's questions will see why:

The Cognitive Questions
(asked by most artists of the 20th century, Platonic or Aristotelian, till around 1958):
"How can I interpret this world of which I am a part? And what am I in it?"

The Postcognitive Questions
(asked by most artists since then):
"Which world is this? What is to be done in it? Which of my selves
is to do it?" (quoted in McHale, 1992, pp. 32–33)

Artists may have begun to look at the world around them in a
new way, but the therapeutic world went on largely unfazed, its
modernist faith intact in the possibility of knowing, loving, and expressing the self as the key to interpreting the world more accurately through finding the self's place in it. The therapeutic agenda was
also quite compatible with the consumer society and its message that
people could find happiness and the affection (and even envy) of
others by gratifying their desires. If people still felt troubled within
by, for instance, guilt or anxiety, psychotherapists were available
to enable the persons to come to terms with themselves, and then
presumably to take their places as productive members of society—
that is, as happy consumers.

The goal for the work of therapy, however it was framed, basically came down to obtaining a better understanding or clearer perception of the world so that a person could find her/his place in it.
It was generally assumed that what stood in the way of accomplishing this goal was the person's unmet "needs," which, since the latter rarely involved the actual necessities of life, tended to mean
unfulfilled desires. These were assumed to distort the person's perception of the world, thereby preventing the person from "getting
in touch with reality." This was part of the modernist agenda of freeing the self from the last of the barriers to its full expression, which
at the psychological level were believed to have their roots in a childhood acceptance of parental injunctions and prohibitions of an ir-
rational and often punitive nature. As a child the person could not
have understood this, but as an adult she/he could; once "knowing
the truth," the person would be "made free" by it.

Developments in Early Family Therapy

When family therapy was invented in the 1950s, it was at first little
more than a variation on psychotherapy. It began slowly, popping

up here and there. On the East Coast, with a psychoanalytic bias, it commenced under the leadership of Nathan Ackerman; quite independently of the latter, though also from a psychoanalytic perspective, Murray Bowen began to explore the influence of families of origin on individuals; and on the West Coast, with a more typically experiential bias, it developed under the charismatic influence of Virginia Satir. Satir's largely atheoretical approach was later supplemented by the provocative ideas of the maverick anthropologist Gregory Bateson, who made the epistemological question explicit. Bateson drew upon the cybernetic thinking that was proliferating hugely by this time, and applied it to an understanding of schizophrenia as a disorder in communication between family members. His ideas were developed and systematized for clinical practice by a highly creative group operating in Palo Alto, comprised of Paul Watzlawick, Don Jackson, Jay Haley, John Weakland, and others. Haley soon went his separate way, abandoning epistemological questions for organizational (and hence bascially ontological) ones; soon, however, another highly charismatic individual, Mara Selvini Palazzoli, heard of the Palo Alto group's work and came to California to study. On her return to Milan, Italy, Selvini Palazzoli and her colleagues Luigi Boscolo, Gianfranco Cecchin, and Giuliana Prata built a highly sophisticated therapeutic methodology out of the cybernetic epistemology of Bateson and his clinical followers. Thus, right into the 1980s, family therapy remained within the modernist tradition, asking, "How can I interpret the world of which I am a part? And what am I in it?"

A variation on late-modernist assumptions characterized the epistemological challenges in the work of the Milan team. Late modernism in literature tends to assume an attitude of suspensive irony, in which judgment is withheld and "the pathos of the modernist hunger for order" has been toned down "to a less anxious acceptance of the world" and its inevitable but manageable disorder (McHale, 1992, p. 22). Late modernism has been typified as "art in a closed field," wherein the conventions of modernism, once so shocking, became predictable. Among the remaining options was a recursive writing of parodic metatexts on nonexistent texts, such as in Vladimir Nabokov's (1962) *Pale Fire* or Jorge Luis Borges's (1961/1964) "Tlon, Uqbar, Orbis Tertius." There is a striking parallel between these practices and the Milan concept of "positive connotation,'' in which, for instance, a family's disorder is paradoxically affirmed in order to free its members of the anxiety that sustains them. The Milan group also approached the family as something of a closed field, which can be best understood to the extent that the therapist team maintains a neutral metaposition to the family. There remained the ironic recognition, however, that no opinion can ever be ''the truth'' about a family, and as such is an invented commentary on the family's own fictions about itself.

Systemic family therapy nudged its way over the imaginary line between late modernism and postmodernism when many champions of the Milan team—Karl Tomm, Paul Dell, and Lynn Hoffman, as well as Boscolo and Cecchin themselves—came under the influence of the brilliant but recondite biologist and ''experimental epistemologist'' Humberto Maturana. Maturana's concepts of ''structural coupling'' and ''structural determinism'' led to the conclusion that no living system can take a metaposition to another. Instead, a process of structural coupling takes place, such that a new system is formed. Maturana's ideas put family therapy at least on the cusp of a postmodern sensibility by acknowledging that since there are no metapositions anywhere in the universe, all we can know are systems in a never-ending process of ''perturbing'' and coupling with one another to form new systems. Furthermore, we can only know what our own biological structures permit us to ''know.'' But since it is our structurally determined capacity for language that even enables us to make such distinctions as systems in the first place, all our perceived ''truths'' are, in the very first instance, constructed ''truths.'' In a sense they are ''true,'' but only in the sense that Richard Rorty suggests we use this word—namely, to honor those distinctions about which a more or less enduring consensus has formed within a community of discourse (Rorty, 1991). Similarly, Maturana's assertion that ''objectivity'' belongs in parentheses resembles Rortys suggestion that it simply refers to a matter about which there is unforced agreement. Not only do such ideas correspond to the postmodern sense that we, in the Western world at least, no longer have either a philosophical or a sociocultural consensus about what constitutes truth; they lead in the direction of an acknowledgment that all we do have are such agreements about the world that people come to through conversation—the world as a construction of common languages.

Recent Innovations

Michael White and his associates, especially David Epston (White & Epston, 1989), have introduced a highly sophisticated sociopolitical vocabulary on the subject of how worlds are constructed that is based to a large extent on Michel Foucault's equation of knowledge and power. White's influence on the field has finally brought family therapy into the postmodern world. In his work he has introduced family therapy to Foucault's neo-Nietzschean writings (cf. Foucault, 1980) on the decentering of the subject and the ubiquity of power pervading all human interaction, such that significant narratives are subjugated to serve the dominant discourse, which comes to define a culture and maintain the status quo. Power operates more like a capillary system that pervades the body than like a sovereign ruling over people. Its role in families, for instance, is at least as effective in maintaining the status quo as is the state itself. Moreover, power is not, as the Enlightenment tradition insisted, banished by knowledge, but vastly increased by it. Power's methods of surveillance and of accumulating information allow it to know all and to see all. As such, it can afford to be benevolent, for it is singularly adept at enlisting the cooperation and even the collaboration of the subjugated in their own subjugation. White's singular genius as a clinician is that he has been able to take this rather bleak vision and apply it to people's everyday lives in the service of their liberation even from such ubiquitous oppression.

White, taking a page from a hitherto overlooked passage in Bateson, says that people do what they do because they are constrained from doing otherwise. The "otherwise" consists in encouraging their access to story lines subjugated by the family's and culture's dominant discourse as to what constitutes the right way of doing things. White's first step in freeing people from their constraints is to separate a person from a problem by "externalizing" the latter. A powerful way of keeping a person in line is to identify him/her with the problem—even when keeping the person in line is not the intention as such. Having people blame themselves is a most powerful way of controlling not only a family, but a populace. Once the problem behavior is separated from the person, it then becomes possible to look for "unique outcomes"—those hitherto neglected or overlooked events or experiences in which the problem has not dominated the person. Once these can be amplified and encouraged, the person (and/or family) is in a position to escape the tyranny of a dominant discourse that has defined him/her as the problem, and hence made the person a docile, self-doubting citizen and consumer.

White's is the first approach to family therapy to begin to embrace the postmodern experience of, in effect, many selves; these selves are viewed, moreover, not as problematic, but as a means of liberation from constraining definitions. White is also the first to view people as custodians of several stories and to see the dominant story as not necessarily in a person's interest—though perhaps in the interests of a more compliant populace. Michael White's friend and colleague David Epston has added to the postmodern direction of current family therapy through his innovation of the "therapeutic letter," in which, in effect, the therapist enters the client's story as a correspondent. The therapist uses the power of carefully crafted language to bring a hitherto subjugated story into the forefront of the client's life; this story replaces a story that is not the client's own, but into which she/he has been recruited.

Vying with White and Epston for breadth of appeal has been the solution-focused therapy of Steve de Shazer and his associates (de Shazer, 1985). There are postmodern elements to this therapy in its independence from foundational theories and its take-it-as-it-comes pragmatism. It also contains postmodern elements in its attention to the "exceptions to the rule"—its insistence that there is a separate life (separate selves, as it were) from the problem-saturated person or family that presents for treatment. Solution-focused therapy is more late-modernist, however, in its apparent faith in technique, which seems to be regarded as applicable to virtually any psychological or interactional problem—and in very short order, to boot. The almost glib assurance that there is a solution to be found is quite at odds with the postmodern temper, with its attitude of modesty and irony in the face of a growing realization that master plans and techniques are no longer so effective in finding a fit for the incommensurabilities of the human situation, large or small.

Postmodern Challenges to Family Therapy

Michael White, perhaps more than any other family therapist, has introduced the narrative dimension—so much a part of postmodern discourse, whether in literary criticism, philosophy, theology, or psychotherapy—into family therapy. This is a signal contribution, to be sure, but in our view White's use of narrative does not make use of the unique implications of work with families, particularly for the postmodern dimensions of the story. Parry (1991a) has tried to address this omission by suggesting that in a radically pluralistic world, everyone has his/her own story *and* participates in the stories of each family member, as well as of each person with whom he/she has significant contact. Parry has also sought to bring the richness and full challenge of the postmodern sensibility more fully into family therapy discourse and clinical practice. To do so, he has suggested that the best source material is to be found not in the ideologically informed pessimism of Foucault and Derrida, but in those who, like therapists, live their professional lives in the domain of stories. Writers and therapists both deal with people interacting with one another amidst the shards of a world in which there is no single binding center, but in which, instead of "things falling apart," they seem to be imploding into one another. The explosion that was modernity, in which all the ancient and traditional connections between people were loosened until all that was left was *self*-expression, has exhausted its explosive power. It is now as if all the loosened pieces, individuals and groups, are collapsing on one another. There is no place to hide from one another, but fewer and fewer common languages with which to speak. The term "postmodern," in short, covers those conditions in contemporary life that confuse so many of the people and families therapists see—the world so well illustrated by the "Zone" in Pynchon's (1973) *Gravity's Rainbow*. In the chaos of the Zone, almost anything goes, the old rules no longer pertain, "an old order is dying and a new one struggling to be born"; people from different worlds speaking different languages mix with one another, and the only way to survive is by making what Pynchon calls "local arrangements" with one another.

For family therapists in particular, this is also the world of the contemporary family. The family is a *crossroads* more than a self-contained *system;* in it a minimum of two generations and two genders come together, depending on one another more than the members often care to admit, even though the generations and the genders more and more frequently inhabit different worlds and speak bafflingly different languages. They may even use the same words, but these may have vastly different meanings. "You used to know what these words mean,'' says the narrator of *Gravity's Rainbow* to the inevitably misreading reader (Pynchon, 1973, p. 472). He could as easily have been talking to the parents of today's teenagers—and not only parents of teenagers, in fact! Today's thoroughly ''Nintendoed'' preadolescent children, who may still be reasonably attentive and even acceptably compliant to the requests and demands of their parents, are growing up with a sensorium attuned to an altogether different world than that of their parents. It is interesting that the best-known of the so-called ''cyberpunk'' writers, William Gibson, who coined the term ''cyberspace'' for that world in which the computer terminal interfaces with the nervous system of its operators, got the idea for the term from video arcade games and computer graphics programs (McHale, 1992, p. 251). Are our children already living in cyberspace?

The phenomenon of ''different worlds, different languages'' is also a product of the demarginalization of people who have been able to find voices of their own and carve out a sense of identity for themselves in the wake of the death of God—the loss of a consensual belief in one single truth. That ''single vision,'' as William Blake called it, is the same drive toward understanding all things ultimately as the Same, which has been identified by Emmanuel Levinas (1991) as the central force in Western thought since Plato. It is, moreover, the same force that Luce Irigaray (1991) identifies as the central patriarchal drive to minimize humans' dependency upon their mortal bodies and upon their mother, the earth—and hence the male dependency upon women. This force's gradual loss of authority in the explosion of modernity has meant that, as Parry (1991a) has suggested earlier, there is no longer an effective or credible margin in place with which to set off those who are the Same (mostly white, heterosexual, European males), aligned with *the* one truth, from those who are Other, different. As peoples who have hitherto been designated Other—women, people of various colors, former colonials, those of homoerotic orientation, even teenagers—begin to speak out and identify themselves with their own stories, they are no longer content to remain marginal characters in the dominant story. They create their own worlds of meaning for themselves and speak their own languages within those worlds.

Is all this another Tower of Babel, or a new Pentecost? To vast numbers, among them many who come to family therapists, it must seem more like the former. Many seem to respond to the cacophony of the postmodern world by seeking a place of stillness, of their own sameness, in a community that shares a familiar story. Many of these are simply parents who cling to the understandable hope that at least their own family can be a place of stability, where their own children at least, respect them enough to comply with their requests, and will grow up under their tutelage to be happy and successful adults. Many family therapists, in turn, perhaps still assume that a family is a more or less coherent "system" that has temporarily over- or undercorrected itself in reaction to some perturbation, and needs only a series of discreetly placed interventions to get back on track as a healthy system again. The very concept of a system, in fact, may be little more than a late-modernist counterpart of the individual self, applied to families. If, as we suggest, however, the family is now more like a crossroads that a system, it may require the services of an interpreter rather than those of a cybernetician.

This shift reflects the move described by Higgins (as quoted by McHale, 1992; see above) from predominantly epistemological questions of how we can *know* the world and our place in it to more ontological questions of what world (or worlds) we *exist* in, what we can do, and which self is to do it. For family therapy this shift has come rather late. The question of how we come to know, as posed by the late modernists Bateson and the Milan group, has shifted to questions of whether we can truly *know* anything, given that our perceptions and assumptions are so strongly influenced by which stories we choose to believe. Once family therapy "went political" and began to listen to the hitherto colonialized (and hence homogenized) voice of arguably the most important person in the family, the mother, the door was opened for the social-constructivist contributions of Marx and Nietzsche, especially as rendered through the writings of Foucault. As salutary as this has been in many ways, it has, in our view, unwittingly embraced a kind of neofoundational privileging of one voice over others: the feminist voice. Since the latter is usually one that speaks for humanity as a whole in a spirit of egalitarianism, it has tended to provide a long-overdue corrective—as long as this is kept in mind and not mistaken for a new "truth."

Because this tendency to privilege the feminist voice has had a tendency to imply that some truths are still truer than others, it has slowed down a recognition of full implications of what families face in a postmodern world—namely, the challenges of raising and living in a family in a world in which no one's perception of reality is intrinsically more accurate than anyone else's. It is a world in which every perception of reality, of one another, and of oneself—including those of the therapist, including this assertion itself—is but an act of interpretation. No person, no theory, no point of view has privilege at the expense of anyone else's. One may, of course, *choose* to give privilege to a particular position—for instance, as, a matter of justice—but that is a (predominantly) ethical decision, not either an epistemological or an ontological statement.

A THERAPY EQUAL
TO THE POSTMODERN CHALLENGES

A therapy equal to the postmodern challenges we have described will have to forsake the temptation of taking the last remaining vestiges of an "objective" or "neutral" position that assumes there is still some piece of firm ground upon which to stand. Most of us therapists are sufficiently informed and sensitive by now to have received this message. But are we yet bold enough to proceed into the postmodern Zone without any security blanket—not even the moral superiority provided by at least an implicit assumption that a particular point of view or way of working *is* just a little bit better or truer than the others? In a word, are we prepared to work entirely within the rather humble acknowledgment that in the intersubjective and even the intrasubjective realm in which therapy takes place, *all* is interpretation?

As such, we work exclusively within the discipline of "hermeneutics." (We might well call our field, in fact, "clinical hermeneutics.") This is a rather lofty word that had its modern beginnings in German theology, where it lived a very active life for well over a century and a half since it was introduced as a major operating principle by the great philosophical theologian Friedrich Schleiermacher. It is simply the science of interpretation, whose reigning deity is Hermes—originally the Greek god of boundaries and roadways, who eventually became the messenger and interpreter from the gods to the human world. Schleiermacher was the first to propose that, whereas common sense operates on the assumption that understanding arises naturally and misunderstanding is an aberration to be overcome, the "more rigorous practice proceeds on the assumption that misunderstanding arises naturally and that understanding must be intended and sought at each point" (quoted in Gadamer, 1976, p. xiii). As such, acccording to Hans-Georg Gadamer—with Paul Ricoeur, probably the foremost exponent of philosophical hermeneutics today—the latter is an ontological discipline, which examines the fundamental and inescapable conditions of living that underlie our efforts to understand. In doing so, it regards understanding as "an event over which the interpreting subject does not ultimately preside" (Gadamer, 1976, p. xi).

People probably come to family therapy in response to problems they are having in understanding one another. They are apt, however, to see their therapsits as individuals who will help them reach a point where they do understand one another, as a result of which the problems in behavior that are generally understood to have arisen as a consequence will be alleviated. In this sense, the epistemological hangover from modernism remains—namely, the assumption that with understanding, with knowing, comes freedom. What would happen, then, it therapists themselves were to adopt the position that not only is it impossible for one person ever to fully understand himself/herself (much less another person), but that this inability extends to therapists as well?

Hermeneutics began with the textual study of the Bible in an effort to get past the inevitable misreading involved in attempting to understand a text that is anywhere from 1,800 to 3,000 years old and was written in a context that is quite alien to the contemporary reader. Today, we are driven to interpret one another's differentness by the demise of those stories that virtually an entire civilization once shared and considered itself a part of, regardless of individuals' generation, gender, color, class, or nationality. There are not only fewer and fewer stories that cross these boundaries, but the boundaries themselves have been more frequently closed off at the very same time as the members of different groups have trouble escaping one another in such a crowded world. The demarginalization of the various groups once defined as the Other, and their accompanying celebratory sharing of stories and a bit of understandable "in your face" attitudinizing, thus far also seem to intensify the inevitability of misreading between those who celebrate difference and those who still value sameness. Moreover, a degree of focus on the self to the neglect of the other often leads to the assumption that others should understand me or us and my or our "needs," but less often to the reverse assumption.

First-order cybernetics teaches us that we can never escape from the limitations of our own perspective, while second-order cybernetics makes it clear that we can never even escape the influence of the perspectives and actions of whatever system we attempt to observe. The introduction of the narrative dimension into family therapy through the work of White and Epston (1989), Goolishian and Anderson (1988), Hoffman (1990), and Parry (1991a), to name only a few, has taken the theme of the limits of perspective a step further. It emphasizes that whether the viewer is a person, a family, a community, or a people, the world is unavoidably viewed through the lens of a succession of stories—not only a personal story, but gender, community, class, and cultural stories. Moreover, if narrative is truly fundamental to the way humans organize and give meaning to experience, it would probably be fair to say that an event only becomes an experience by being narrated. This corresponds to the sense in which Fredric Jameson (1981) describes narrative, as "the central function or *instance* of the human mind" (p. 13; emphasis Jameson's). As such, narrative is not simply a new way of doing therapy, one bound to be replaced after we tire of asking people to "tell me your story." In short, we cannot *not* do narrative therapy.

When we say with Jameson that narrative is "the central function or *instance* of the human mind," and that it is necessarily the language of therapy, we are also saying that it is the master code by which a person interprets the text of her/his life in order to give it meaning. But since a person's life connects with the lives of so many others, her/his stories are, more precisely, the code according to which the person deciphers the meaning of life as text. "Text" is a quintessentially postmodernist term, as "Work" was for modernism. It replaces the modernist term by regarding objects or persons as "immense ensembles or systems of texts . . . superimposed on each other by way of the various intertextualities, successions of fragments [such that the] automomous work of art thereby—along with the old autonomous subject or ego—seems to have vanished, to have been volatilized" (Jameson, 1991, p. 77). Is something like this not what we work with in the demise of those unifying metanarratives that formerly pulled everything together to create a single meaning—or a single self?

Metanarratives were the means used by people to decode personal and local narratives in an almost allegorical sense; in this process, according to Jameson, "the data of one narrative line are radically impoverished by their rewriting according to the paradigm of another narrative, which is taken as the former's master code or Ur-narrative and proposed as the ultimate hidden or unconscious meaning of the first one'' (1981, p. 22). Thus an individual person's life might, in effect, be subject to decoding according to the Christian master code. In the demise of all grand narratives, we now live in a world in which personal narratives essentially stand alone as the means by which we pull together the text of our own lives, as well as the "intertextual" overlappings of those lives that enter ours. Although this may all be frightening without the legitimating guidance of the grand narratives, it is also a liberating possibility. It frees us from the totalizing tyranny of the grand narratives, however benign most of them might have been. Our own stories stand alone as the codes according to which we interpret the significance and meaning of the text of our own lives and of those others who concern us. There is no longer a mediating code between our own personal narratives and the lives which our stories are trying to make sense of. The narrative thread with we elect to identify ourselves is the only code we have any longer for that purpose, and only to the extent that we *intentionally* embrace such stories as our own.

Meanwhile, beyond the person-to-person level, the large impersonal forces in the postindustrial world of state and corporate powers are at last unhampered by any requirement that they be held to account by the canons of a grand narrative that morally legitimizes their enterprises. They no longer operate in the narrative domain at all. Their activities are self-legitimizing on the basis of the principle of "performativity"—of continuing to do what they already do, and doing it efficiently with no regard whatever for metaphysical or metanarrative considerations. Giant systems operate by their own self-generated procedures, which operate in the interests of getting things done to insure their own perpetuation. Individuals and their various personal narratives are no match against these vast forces, which attend to them only "to make individuals 'want' what the system needs in order to perform well" (Lyotard, 1984, p. 62). (The one area in which narrative does continue to play a significant, shaping role within the corporate world is the realm of entertainment. Here, stories are transmitted to a degree never before possible; moreover, they appeal to the yen for instant gratification, quick resolution, and fantasy indulgence in which a consumer society is deeply entrenched.) This state of affairs contributes to a continuing sense of passivity and powerlessness, which probably accounts for much of the appeal of narratives of victimhood.

The postmodern world also poses an unprecedented challenge to family life. There is no legitimizing metanarrative that intrinsically gives the family any more than the individual a special claim on the lives of its members, or parents authority over their children. Family members, even the youngest, leave the family daily and return bearing new and strange narratives—the children from their peers and from their schooling; the parents from their jobs and coworker interactions, their gender affiliations, and their recreational peer associations. The parents' parents bring in turn, from their associations with their own generation, stories intensified by a lifetime of ways of interacting with their adult children, as well as values they may now be wishing to pass on through their stories to their grandchildren. On top of all this, more and more families are mixtures of multiple marriages and relationships with children from each.

In short, the contemporary family is, as never before, a crossroads in which its different members go forth to and return from different worlds where different languages are spoken, different stories are told, and different selves are employed. Every vestige of the world of unities is under attack. In the face of this, the only recourse parents have in dealing with the problems their children face in coping with the only world they have ever known are the stories they bring out of their own experiences; these, like all such small narratives, entirely lack authority. What can family therapy offer families in a world in which neither the family as an institution, nor the parents as individuals, have any reliable consensual moral authority to draw upon?

WHAT NARRATIVE CAN STILL DO

If narrative is intrinsically the language of therapy, is there yet hope in the power of narrative, when it lacks authority, to lift people's lives and bring them together again? In a world that lacks a legitimizing yardstick against which to measure one's own and others' lives, certain features become apparent. One is that each person's stories become self-legitimizing. A story told by a person in his/her own words of his/her own experience does not have to plead its legitimacy in any higher court of narrative appeal, because no narrative has any greater legitimacy than the person's own. Therefore, attempts by others to question the validity of such a story are themselves illegitimate. They are coercive, and to the extent that such methods are used to silence or discredit a person's stories, they represent a form of terrorism. We use such a strong word advisedly, for when one person tries to silence the legitimate voice of another, this is done invariably by throwing into question that person's only resource for discerning reality, her/his own judgment. All those who are thrown into that position of self-doubt are being thrown out of their own stories and robbed of their own voices.

The first major task for a postmodern family therapy, therefore, becomes that of encouraging people in the legitimizing of their own stories. This involves reminding them that there are no other yardsticks of stories or persons against which to measure the legitimacy of their own stories. The second task is that of encouraging people to appreciate that when they use their *own* words to describe their *own* experiences, no one has any right to take the legitimacy of that story away from them under any circumstances. A story is a person's own story, and he/she is its poet. Richard Rorty says:

> To fail as a poet, and thus, for Nietzsche, to fail as a human being is to accept somebody else's description of oneself, to execute a previously prepared program, to write, at most, elegant variations on previously written poems. *So the only way to trace home the causes of being as one is would be to tell a story about one's causes in a new language.* (1989, p. 28; emphasis added)

Third, when there is no central story against which to evaluate that of either an individual or a family, then, not only do all persons' and all families' ways of being themselves through the stories they tell become self-legitimizing, but each person is freed from the assumption that a grand narrative tends to foster—namely, that each person is entitled to only one self. In a time of different worlds and different languages, different selves will be called upon to perform the many different deeds expected of people in their different worlds.

Still another task of the present-day narrative family therapist is to help each person liberate the many stories that have been censored into oblivion by the tyranny of a single, dominant story—one, moreover, that has been falsely identified as *the* self. Michael White was the first to look for what he has called "unique outcomes": those

lost stories (lost because not noticed, and hence not told about individuals and families) in which the offending problem is solved, or
not even encountered. One of the primary dividends of the postmodern eclipse of the grand narratives is the overthrow of the tyranny
of the One and the Same. Thus no one need be held to account by
a single, dominant sequence of similar stories. People are free to pick
and choose by which sequence of stories they wish to be known and
remembered. Walt Whitman (1855/1959) sang:

> Do I contradict myself?
> Very well, I contradict myself.
> (I am large, I contain multitudes.) (p. 68)

Before people can be free to choose which of their multitude of
stories they wish to be identified with, it is therapeutically imperative that they be freed from the tyranny of those stories lurking behind the story of frustration that families and individuals bring to
therapy. The great contribution of Jacques Derrida and deconstruction to family therapy has been—aside from reminding us that this
is what therapists have been doing, at least since Freud—to call our
attention to the fact that no story or text stands alone. Behind every story is another story. Thus, in any complaint that a family brings
to a therapist involving a recurring cycle of behavior—what Tomm
(1991) calls a "pathologizing interactional pattern"—we find that
it is well to inquire about the story behind that story. When people
use the popular expression of "pushing each other's buttons," we
suggest that those "buttons" will invariably be connected to the painful memory of a story associated with each person's sense of having
had to struggle for psychological survival. Each old story is what gives
the current "stuck story" its driving urgency. Nor is it enough simply to identify an old story as the "reason" a person is currently
behaving so defensively. That connection has been used all too frequently either to accuse or pathologize the other, or to excuse the
self. The old story, rather, is best brought forth in graphic detail and
shown to each person as one in which a struggle for psychological
survival was at stake. The therapeutic goal is not to supply reasons
or offer explanations, but to awaken compassion in each toward the
other and toward the self.

Liberated from the wishful modernist fiction that the soul of a
person, like that of any object of scientific scrutiny, can be fully

known, postmodern narrative therapists and their clients need not get caught up in the futile and self-defeating task of trying to ''get it right.'' The more we face and acknowledge the plurality of persons and perspectives in the postmodern world, the more we are brought up against the unfathomable mystery of the human imagination, the author of all stories. Under the tyranny of one dominant story, and hence of one ruling self, it seemed possible and even desirable to know oneself and to understand the other. Once we begin to realize how many stories and thus how many selves we are capable of encompassing, we start to grasp the fact that all our ''readings'' of others and of ourselves are bound to be ''misreadings.'' After all, we only perceive others through our own stories, and ourselves through that same self-magnifying lens. We can come to see, therefore, that difficulties with ourselves and others are the results of ''negative misreadings'' of our own or others' intentions, or both. When we react to an anticipated negative misreading, we invariably invite a corresponding negative misreading in reaction, and the interchange enters the realm of self-fulfilling prophecies. Negative misreadings are best reversed, but not by a ''more accurate'' reading. They are best reversed by a ''compassionate misreading''—a decision to interpret the actions of the other as, in Rorty's term, a ''fellow sufferer.'' That is, we can conclude that an offending other is likely to be acting more out of anxiety, hurt, or confusion than out of meanness, perversity, or dislike of us. There is always the chance that such an interpretation will be wrong, but the *performative* consequences are still more likely to be beneficial than those proceeding from a negative misreading.

Finally, the postmodern family therapist of narrative persuasion is well advised to remain mindful of the fact that a family's members will continue to be subjected to the influences of the different worlds and different languages that prevail today; thus, the family itself can no longer be assumed to be strong enough in its binding power to exert the kinds of influence that parents feel necessary to withstand these influences. Narrative family therapists have a very important role to play in assisting families in finding ways of making their members feel connected meaningfully and pleasurably to one another. No bond today responds very well to the imperative of what ''should'' be. In our view, every cultural institution and community that endures is held together by the stories its members share with one another (Parry, 1991b). Families have been thought of for countless millennia as places where stories were shared in the normal course of events. In today's crossroads family, this once-spontaneous practice can readily be lost—particularly as members relate to one another with criticism and recrimination on the one hand, and efforts to free themselves from old dependencies on the other. The encouragement of rituals that invite the sharing of stories among family members can become a powerful means of strengthening family ties, passing on important values, and developing a family world and language again in its own right as a rival to the plurality of loyalties that otherwise can make of today's family a postmodern Tower of Babel.

Narrative, then, continues to have much to offer, even in a postmodern world that lacks legitimizing metanarratives. As therapists, we continue to deal with the stories people tell us about the disordering of the text of their lives. By regarding these stories as interpretations of this text that keep resulting in unhappy experiences, we can help them in our conversations to find more satisfying interpretations by bringing forth stories that are more congruent with the lives they intend to live. Each such text is the story of someone's efforts to live in this Zone called the postmodern world, in which, in the collapse of common rules or stories, we can only hope to be able to make "arrangements" with one another through our inescapable participation in one another's stories. As each person expands that sense of participation to embrace all life—that is to say, every being capable of suffering—each can develop her/his own metanarrative.

POSTMODERN ETHICS
AND THE MYSTERY OF THE OTHER

A personal metanarrative would play the role metanarratives have always played: calling forth responsibility toward the Other, or, in other words, addressing the ethical domain. The Other played a central role in the legitimizing role of the dominant sacred story, in its imperatives to "love thy neighbor as thyself" and to "do unto others as you would have them do unto you." It was also present in those metanarratives inspired by the 18th-century Enlightenment. However, psychotherapy, that quintessential modernist creation, placed the feelings and "needs" of the self ahead of obligations toward the Other, because individuals felt particularly constrained by the demands of a moribund morality that insisted they despise themselves but love their fellow human beings. The success of the modern market economy, moreover, has been built upon convincing consumers that their happiness lies in self-gratification.

The historic grand narratives held Western society together in some sense of "us-ness," in spite of the centrifugal forces of modernity. It is their demise that has left us living in different worlds, speaking different languages; even groups seem content to serve their own members, but to display indifference to most others. Thus the very process that has increasingly liberated the hitherto marginalized Other from a tyranny exercised by many of the grand narratives, especially the sacred ones, has created, in some cases, new "us against them" attitudes. It is this movement, however, that has brought the question of the Other into the forefront of European (though not, curiously enough, Anglo-American) thought.

As the postmodern world moves more and more in the direction of pluralization, multiculturalism, or even a planetary civilization, difference rather than sameness becomes the order of things and the Other becomes the ethical challenge of the present. The two continental philosophers who have most eloquently made responsibility toward the Other the cornerstone of an ethic for our time are Emmanuel Levinas (1991) and Luce Irigaray (1991). Levinas came to France from a Lithuanian Jewish background; Irigaray is a psychoanalyst who was banished from membership in the Lacanian *école freudienne* and from her teaching position upon the publication of her book *Speculum of the Other Woman* in 1974. Levinas addressed the matter of the Other in a sweeping critique of Western philosophical thought since Plato, from the point of view of the Biblical prophetic tradition that recalls each person to the Other's absolute claim of responsibility upon him/her. Western thought has involved a quest for a universal truth. As such, it has privileged the Same over the Other, the different, seeking to rein the latter into the former in the interests of the ideal of universality. The result of this has been that the Other has been given no ontological status. Levinas seeks nothing less than to reverse 2,500 years of philosophy and language by privileging instead the Other over the Same. "I am trying to show," he says, "that man's ethical relation to the other is ultimately prior to his ontological relation to himself (egology) or the the totality of things that we call the world (cosmology)" (Levinas & Kearney,

1974/1986, p. 21). He goes on: "My ethical relationship of love for the other stems from the fact that the self cannot survive by itself alone, cannot find meaning within its own being-in-the-world, within the ontology of sameness" (1974/1986, p. 21).

Irigaray takes Levinas a crucial step further, identifying the imperialism of the Same with the domination of the male and the subordination of women. The universal truth of the spirit as aspiration involved the subordination and escape from matter, the dark realm of the mother/woman. Women henceforth were denied the status of subjects and became instead the objects of male exchange, just as the material, feminine earth became a commodity available for the exploitation and domination of (the) man. For Irigaray, the primordial crime, then, was not the Oedipal patricide, but matricide.

Only when woman as Other is embraced fully in her difference from the imperial sameness of male phallocracy will it become possible to fully demarginalize everything and every people who have been fitted into that historic servant/slave role of Other. Only then will the Other be able to be embraced just *because*, not in spite of, being different from oneself. Levinas envisions in almost messianic fashion the possibility as an ethical imperative of the "face-to-face" meeting with the Other whose difference is cherished rather than overcome. Irigaray is also visionary. She writes of the "divinity of love," the "amorous exchange," and the "sensible transcendent" in which the love of two human beings is metaphorical for the experience of God; the relation of body to body is an image for the surrender of boundaries (Irigaray, 1986).

It was inevitable, given the historic context, that psychotherapy had to relativize moral questions in order to liberate individuals from their often irrationally guilt-inducing constraints. Family therapy, by contrast, is obliged to seek an ethical stance. In families, the Other is always present as challenge and opportunity. This is particularly so in a world in which there is no limit on the desire of individuals for their own aggrandizement. Yet when family members tell their stories to one another, each is granted a glimpse into the sheer mystery of another person. When the members then use their imaginations and relate the others' told experiences to themselves, the sharing of stories can provide a bridge of compassion across which that mystery can be, in those moments, breached, and hitherto alienating differences can be found to contain similarities in one of each member's own multitude of stories. In a time of different worlds and different languages, an ethic that calls each of us to embrace the differences in our loved ones, the differences in the strangers in our midst, and even the differences in ourselves may, through the stories we share, be able to serve as a life-enhancing craft afloat on an otherwise uncharted world/ocean.

OLD STORIES AND THEIR RE-VISION

The Importance of Childhood Models: The Neurobiological Basis

When Freud's "children" began to challenge their "father," they did so on the issue of his claim of the refractory role played by childhood experiences in determining adult behavior. For Alfred Adler, the childhood inferiority complex could be overcome through awakening a person's inherent social feeling. For C. G. Jung, the imbalances induced from early experiences could be redressed by the balancing and teleological operations of the collective unconscious. Otto Rank, the first "brief therapist," wanted to cut through the traumas of childhood to tackle the birth trauma as a prototype of all subsequent separation anxieties by encouraging the person's "courage to will." The neo-Freudians, led by Karen Horney, sought to address the presenting issues in the present rather than the past. Horney's example has been enthusiastically followed by most nonmedical therapists, from Carl Rogers through the behaviorists to Steve de Shazer and his solution-focused school today.

We also prefer a brief approach to therapy, but maintain that the emphasis on childhood as the source of later difficulties for individuals and families alike is inescapable and has a very basic explanation. Its roots go back to our prehistoric past, which has left its mark in our genetic code. In their excellent survey and application to psychotherapy of the findings of evolutionary psychologists and biologists, Kalman Glantz and John Pearce (1989) state, on the basis of neurobiological evidence, that one of the primary functions of the brain is to create a "model" of the world—a kind of internal road map designed to help the otherwise helpless child survive. They write:

> The creative power of the cortex is a two-edged sword. It makes it
> possible for humans to generate models of magnificent complexi-

ty, but also makes it possible to form models that are self-defeating
and/or destructive to others. . . . In a confusing environment, a perfectly good brain can generate a perfectly terrible model. (p. 10)

Particularly because human beings are uniquely vulnerable and
equipped with few of the instinctual resources possessed by other
animals, the ''autocatalytic'' growth in the size of the brain during
the past 2 million years appears to have developed in order to provide our ancestors with a capacity to respond to novel circumstances
with a prepared strategy. Probably all highly developed mammals
possess to some degree a neurologically based model of their world.
None, however, comes even close to our human capacity to model
reality with the adaptive capacity and sheer complexity that our brains
make possible.

According to Richard Alexander (1989), this development of the
brain has had more to do with adapting to the complexities of the
human social environment than adapting to the biophysical demands
imposed by hunting, gathering, avoiding predatory beasts, and con-
triving clothing and shelter which were the primary survival activities of our forerunners. Humans lived in groups in which the males
hunted wild animals for meat and the females gathered roots, fruits,
and nuts. The population of humans was small; unless there was
a scarcity of resources in certain areas, groups might have been expected to have to compete with other groups or bands relatively in-
frequently. There does seem to be evidence that our early ancestors
were highly cooperative within their familiar groups of families and
band members, but were intensely competitive and very aggressive
toward members of other bands, particularly when territories over-
lapped or resources were scarce. A complicating factor where such
competition was concerned was a pronounced tendency to treat competing bands of other humans as if they were of a different species
of predators. As such, the other groups would end up being treated
in ways in which the norms applying to fellow band members did
not apply. This may have been the origin of that ominous
phenomenon—the categorization of strangers, slaves and scapegoats
as Other, and hence less human.

Life, at any rate, was very basic for our forebears; yet it must
have been sufficiently complex at the social level, even within the
band, to have given rise to the development of a vast brain capable
of a high degree of consciousness, including the processing of the

emotions, thoughts, plans, imagination, insight, foresight, memory, deception, self-deception, intentions, self-image, and language. Alexander suggests that this complexity as an aid to survival may have arisen initially as a resource for the young, with its extension into adulthood as a fortunate spillover. Humans are an intensely social species, and a higher degree of complexity than might first meet the eye is involved in learning all the "rules" of interaction that are necessary to adapt successfully to living together in groups. Social learning involves especially learning the rules of reciprocity—the balancing of favors, and the remembering and tallying of slights and hurts. It was probably vital that a child begin to learn these rules from a very young age in order to survive in the band and the tribe. Nicholas Humphrey (1976) observes:

> Social primates are required by the very nature of the system they create and maintain to be calculating beings; they must be able to calculate the consequences of their own behavior, to calculate the likely behavior of others, to calculate the balance of advantage and loss—and all this in a context where the evidence on which their calculations are based is ephemeral, ambiguous, and liable to change, not least as a consequences of their own actions. (p. 19)

The uniquely lengthy period of childhood dependency upon adults is especially valuable at this point. There is much to learn about the intricacies of the world to which children must learn to adapt, but fortunately they are given a generous period of time in which to learn it, and a protective environment in which to practice. Protection and preparation in a sense equal play, and our ancient forebears placed a great deal of emphasis on play as the basis for learning. For them, play was, in effect, practice for survival. In the course of such protected learning, children quickly began, then as now, to build in what Bateson (1972) and other cyberneticians many years ago began calling "maps." Glantz and Pearce (1989), as mentioned earlier, refer to a "model" of the universe, while Alexander (1989) refers to built-in "scenarios" for reality testing. To the extent that such models or scenarios correspond to subsequent challenges, they no longer simply serve as makeshift guides. They become "reality itself," and, particularly when a person is anxious, may take precedence over the actual obstacles that the person is about to face. It is as if the brain makes a program of the world in early life, and once this is accomplished simply rejects or at most reinterprets any incoming information that is at odds with the program, to make it fit the program rather than vice versa—particularly if survival is deemed at stake. In such an instance, rapid reaction is imperative; there may not be time for the luxury of waiting and seeing, or additional reality testing. This, we propose, is the reason why many childhood models appear to be so firmly incorporated that they resist persuasion, exhortation, or even contrary evidence: They have been formed on the basis of partial data, amidst the apprehension that the challenge at hand involves survival. Accordingly, the model is cemented in as reality itself. Until modified, the power of the resulting story of the world is such that it will keep the person looking backward for direction, as it were, rather than facing forward to meet what is coming.

Emotions as Narrative Constructs

The human brain, in short, may have the property of forming cognitive maps, but it seems to be much less effective in altering or undoing the parameters of such a map one it has been identified as *the* map of "reality." In fact, the capacity to form intentions, often in order to change the reality that people themselves have mapped, is frequently frustrating precisely because the world as programmed tends, then, to override the conscious intention. It is probably this phenomenon that Freud designated as the unconscious. But, lest all of this sound a mite deterministic and fixed, and we be accused of the dread postmodern heresy of "essentialism" or, worse yet, "foundationalism" let us be clear that our position at this point is rooted in two aspects of human life that we suggest are simply irreducible. The first is the inescapable *embodiedness* of human life, and the history of its evolution that is carried in human bodies through the DNA text. The second is that what people construct through language and narrative are *meanings*, not natural phenomena. These two features represent the interface between the materiality of the earth and the sociality of the world. For Heidegger, "the work of art emerges in the gap between Earth and World, or what I would prefer to translate as the meaningless materiality of the body and nature and the meaning endowment of history and of the social" (quoted in Jameson, 1991, p. 7). It is to bridge this gap that human beings have made up stories.

Moreover, storytelling as means of making the world is undoubtedly with us from birth for we are born into a storied world and are assigned parts to play even before we draw our first breath. Our embodiedness and our sociality, then, give us what Heidegger called a sense of being "thrown" into existence, beset by certain givens. Thus, children enter the world equipped with a genetic heritage that they did not ask for, as either boys or girls, born into families that were not requested. They then find themselves identified as characters in the stories of their parents and siblings, as well as in an entire family tradition of tales about members. At the same time, the children themselves are hard at work with the advent of the self-consciousness that language makes possible, inventing stories for themselves that both will make sense of the world in which they find themselves and will serve as guides for responding to the significant others of their lives, in order to survive in a world of giants. We can deny as many of these givens as we like, although if we have learned anything from Freud, it should be that we ignore anything unpalatable about ourselves at our own—and often the world's—peril.

Phyllis Nussbaum (1988) also suggests, in a very arresting article, that our emotions themselves represent nothing less than "the acceptance of, the assent to live according to, a certain sort of story. Stories, in short, contain and teach forms of feeling, forms of life" (p. 218). Nussbaum roots her argument in three famous novels of Samuel Beckett (*Malone, Malone Dies, The Unnamable*). These novels imaginatively propose that liberation from such emotions as fear, guilt, disgust, hope, and love can be obtained only by escaping from the stories that have conditioned them. Once people are outside these shaping stories, subsequent experiences no longer elicit those emotions. Emotions, then, are not natural stirrings, but narrative constructs. Once constructed, however, they cannot be simply willed away. The stories in which they are embedded have to be deconstructed and decoded to yield the stubborn beliefs about "reality" to which emotions are reactions.

Beckett's target is the narrative that has most shaped and conditioned the way people react in Western culture: the Christian story of humanity's fall into sin and guilt, and the possibility of attaining redemption, love, and happiness through self-denial and suffering. For Beckett, that story not only creates and sustains those emotions in people; its shaping power informs all subsequent cultural, familial, and personal stories. His answer to its monolithic tyranny is to escape the influence of stories altogether, and thereby to discover ''that the world does not need to be interpreted, it can simply be lived in, accepted, trusted as the birds trust'' (Nussbaum, 1988, p. 238). But, as Nussbaum wryly points out, this is simply another story. For the storytelling animal, the only alternative to stories is silence.

The Construction of Childhood Survival Stories

If the stories into which children are born create and shape their emotions, they do so by constructing what the children *believe* to be real. We suggest that in addition to being inescapably born into an already storied world, children actively enter these stories as soon as they equip themselves with a language, continuing them as a means of making them their own reality. As such they become the children's truth, their world. The more, however their very survival seems threatened by abusive actions, threats, perceptions, or experiences of abandonment, the more rigidly incorporated such stories become. When a child's world-shaping stories come to imply risks to his/her survival, they include two significant messages: ''This is what you must *avoid* to survive'' (either physically or psychologically) and ''This is what you can *do* to survive—and maybe even be loved.''

For most children in modern urban societies, the dangers in the home, where they should be safest, are primarily psychological (although for too great a minority, they are also physical). However, children react to emotional or psychological threats just as protectively as they would to a threat to their physical survival. Indeed, in our opinion—based on our joint clinical experiences, as well as our understandings of the evidence that is accumulating from evolutionary psychology—children are disposed, by virtue of their youthful helplessness, to trust that they can leave the issue of survival in the hands of their parents and extended family members. They use the trust and safety of this environment to practice reality in the form of play and exploration of the boundaries of the world in which they are newcomers. Our hunting and gathering ancestors lived in a dangerous world, but apparently managed to combine protectiveness with a certain permissiveness where learning from controlled experiences was concerned. Accordingly, their children seem to have been raised according to the principle that the family (band) and home are safe and the world beyond is dangerous (Glantz & Pearce, 1989, p. 77). Several thousand generations were raised according to this assumption. Accordingly, we might be justified in assuming that present-day humans, their descendants, are genetically predisposed as children to trust home but mistrust the outside world, until they are informed otherwise. When that predisposition is countered and the children discover that family and home are unsafe it is our contention that their emerging story of the world quickly turns into what we call a "survival story."

Experiences of threat, abuse, or abandonment (actual or perceived) are so at variance with children's embodied predispositions of what to expect that they are programmed into the realm of embodied reactivity reserved for experiences too important to be left to conscious discernment (Alexander, 1989, pp. 491–492). Survival is the primary impulse and first priority. Accordingly, threatened children must be able to avoid at all costs actions and even fantasies that might offend their parents, and at the same time to develop behaviors and attitudes that invite parental approval. In order to make sure that they engage in both of these, the children are likely to remember best stories that portray family members in as favorable a light as necessary. At the same time, dangerous impulses and experiences, the "unspeakable," dare not be spoken. Nonetheless, these continue their influence in the form of unstoried anxious reactions against anything that might interfere with the strategy of responding to the parents in such ways as to obtain approval and escape annihilation. Any threat or prospect of the recurrence of experiences similar to the "unspeakable" events will sufficiently alarm the children that they will automatically try to avoid them, even when, in chaotically abusive families, such efforts prove futile.

Uncovering the Hidden Text

However, when attention is paid to such habituated stylistic cues as tone of voice, reactivity to particular issues or interactions, bodily postures, or facial expressions that are apt to occur as persons or families tell stories of current or past events, clues are dropped and tracks left that are apt to lead back to the dark reality that has shaped the stories themselves. By thus following what we call "the tracks of a hidden text," the persons can be brought back to the "unspeakable'' itself—those experiences whose very existence was denied by a conspiracy of silence that first divested them of their own voices, by which alone they could describe their own experiences in their own words. At this point the individuals can resume the writing and living of their own stories and abdicate from those stories into which they were born and which have defined them and lived them.

The hidden text, in other words, has shaped a survival story made up of heavily expurgated experiences that conspired to these individuals as children this early message: ''If only you will do this or that, I [we] will love you.'' These messages, which are apt to be delivered quite openly, tend to consist of actions and attitudes involving socially acceptable behavior. As such, they may be restricted in some cases to idiosyncratic behaviors acceptable to the parents and family members, pertaining to particular family traditions and preferences. Other messages are apt to involve expectations of conventional social virtues, such as pleasing people, trying hard, being the best, being nice, being emotionally reserved, being emotionally expressive—as many behaviors as there are more or less specific familial and cultural virtues. It does not matter whether the children ever get the promised approval for observing such expected virtues; it only matters that they *believe* that ''if only'' they behave properly, they will receive the desired approval and the assurances of love and emotional safety that are promised.

We must emphasize, however, that when we use terms such as ''survival story'' and ''hidden text,'' they are meant as images that seem to have a powerful metaphorical resonance for those who have grown up in abusive or chaotic families, and who therefore continue to be dogged in their efforts to raise children or even simply to live their lives free of crippling self-doubt. They continue to be constrained by the power of an old story that enabled them to survive what was for them a harrowing childhood, but that is of no value for adult living and for raising reasonably happy families that are free of abusiveness. For those for whom childhood was less harrowing, and a sense of survival as individuals was not so much at stake, the world they formed through the stories they were born into and those they invented to make sense of it very likely continues to hold to them more stubbornly than they may prefer. Their childhood story, in short, does not terrorize them; as a consequence, it does not have to be thrown as radically into question in order for them to be able to live closer to the ways they intend. It may well unduly constrain them, however, and they may seek a story re-vision on that account. The following two clinical vignettes illustrate the difference between the two, but they also suggest the value of an approach that identifies and externalizes an old childhood story in order to free a person of its constraining influence in the present. In one case, the client was living according to a toxic story; in the other, she was living according to a benevolent but now unhelpful story.

Noreen was a woman of 35 who kept finding herself in situations in which her efforts to "do the right thing" invariably climaxed with her defending herself against the abusive reactions of those she was trying to please. The "tracks" of these events led back to a series of abusive experiences, which climaxed in the memory of a time when she had hidden in her parents' bedroom to prepare a surprise for them. When her whereabouts were discovered, her drunk father banged on the door threateningly, forced an entrance, and delivered a fearful beating to the confused and terrified child. Noreen's survival story seemed to be driven by the belief that if only she made angry people happy, they would love her. When their anger seemed merely aggravated rather than appeased, she would blame herself and try yet again, believing that their anger was a result of her failure to appease them. Once this survival story was identified and externalized, it was "exorcised," and Noreen was able to build a new life based on a story of making others happy through looking after her own happiness.

Marcia, on the other hand, had grown up in a very loving and affirming home, which allowed her to create a story of love, kindness, and fairness as the correct and most helpful response to any misunderstanding or mistreatment at the hands of others. When she left a marriage in which her husband had begun to flaunt his new lovers in front of her at social gatherings, his rage seemed to know no bounds. She would respond to his efforts at revenge with unfailing kindness and attempts to explain herself to him. He apeared to react to these by retaliating even more, using especially their children—especially the elder, a boy—as his weapons. Once Marcia began to identify and externalize the sources of her innocence in her childhood story of "a good Catholic girl," she was able to take what she cherished from that story and attach it to a story re-vision of showing love by protecting both her children and herself wherever necessary. She became increasingly confident, and her son, who had become a frighteningly confused adolescent, began to find himself and to make his own choices.

The Process of Story Deconstruction and Re-Vision

In either type of situation, the experiences that bring individuals or families to therapy represent, in our view, a "wake-up call"—a message that the stories that have formed them and shaped their emotional reactions have reached their limit. Although these stories made sense to children dependent upon adults, they are no longer adequate to help the individuals handle present challenges effectively. It is now time for them to question the beliefs and assumptions that their stories have coded, in order to free themselves from the constraints upon capacities that maturity and responsibility have since made available to them. In ancient times going back to the Paleolithic (and even among the few surviving tribal peoples of today), stories that shaped a person as a child were divested of their power through elaborate rituals observed at the dawn of adulthood. These ceremonies were death–rebirth rituals through which the limits of the childhood story were put to death; by means of the often painful rites of passage involved, an adult man or woman was born who was already provided with the intitiating episode of their new story (Eliade, 1958). Today we must do this with therapy, which often does not begin, if it begins even then, until a crisis in our individual or family life strikes with the message that the old story is finished. It is time for story deconstruction and re-vision.

A story deconstruction consists, in essence, of identifying the terms, the shape, and the plot of an individual's childhood survival story—what the person is coming to realize she/he had to do to survive childhood. The person is also invited to regard that child, who did what was necessary to survive. Some children will have had to struggle heroically in the face of physical, sexual, or emotional abuse; others will not have had to struggle so hard, but may have had to limit themselves unduly or shape themselves along very constraining lines. In each case, the therapist invites the person to salute and cherish the strength and wit that enabled her/him to get through her childhood limitations. This person is no victim, but a survivor and more.

Once the shape and plot of the story, and the threads connecting innumerable stories according to an interpretive assumption about the self and the world, are basically identified and recognized, the story can be externalized. Once this is accomplished, various access points into the story are identified. This is done fairly easily. They can be found wherever a person finds himself/herself to be characteristically "reactive"—that is, experiences anxiety, rage, guilt, and/or shame that seem disproportionate to current circumstances. The old story that is still living the person can be externalized as a whole according to those interactions, which can increasingly be recognized as the points of imposition of an old story upon a current situation. The person's reactions to the latter can be identified as unworkable because they come out of a story that has little to offer for the current challenge.

Once an old story is externalized as a once necessary but now unworkable story, steps can be taken to interfere with its reactive urgency by imposing key "stoppers," such as a story-epitomizing mantra (Sheinberg, 1992) or the question "What story is this?". Such techniques will enable a person to establish the basis for a story revision—based no longer on reactions over which she/he feels little control or even responsibility, but upon immediate choices and improvisations. No one ever fully becomes the author of her/his own story; any such assumption can only lead back into the illusions of control, individual autonomy, isolated selfhood, and single truth. The person goes forth instead to join with others in the universal human action of multiple authorship.

CHAPTER 3

Helping People Become Authors of Their Own Stories

In Chapter 2, we have briefly outlined a narrative style of therapy that examines the "survival stories" people construct and are constructed by during childhood and adolescence. In many cases, these stories provided templates for actual physical or psychological survival in threatening situations during childhood; in other instances, the sense of actual survival was less at stake, but the stories provided guidelines for making sense of and coping with the adult world. In either case, a "wake-up call"—that is, a crisis conveying the message that a story is no longer helpful and often actually harmful to an individual or a family—is what brings the person or family to therapy. We have used these concepts to establish a context for the telling of clients' stories, such that those involved in these narratives begin to see them as hermeneutics (i.e., interpretations) rather than as life itself. We should emphasize, however, that there are many other ways of practicing narrative therapy that do not use the "survival story" and "wake-up call" metaphors.

This chapter presents an overview of narrative approaches that are informed by a variety of family systems theories (structural, strategic, systemic, etc.), and that also provide space for the deconstruction of a client's story so that it can be viewed as only one interpretation among many possible ones (both past and present). This is not to suggest that the client's interpretation is trivial; rather, it is one that has been "living the client," actually inhabiting him/her in the form of meanings and views of the world. Once the client is engaged in the process of telling this story in a context where it can be viewed as a highly influential text that he/she did not totally author, the initial work of story deconstruction has begun. As the process of deconstruction is taking place, space for story re-vision is created. In our view, deconstruction and re-vision are not separate processes, but are equally important and inescapably linked. Deconstruction opens space for story re-vision, and re-vision provides the opportunity for further deconstruction. Thus, many of the ideas presented below can be used for both deconstructive and re-visioning purposes. As is true of all the remaining chapters, an end-of-chapter appendix of sample therapeutic questions and dialogues is included to aid readers in experimenting with these concepts in their own work. The item numbers in the appendix correspond to those in the text proper.

THE IMPORTANCE OF STORY RE-VISION

The importance of the re-vision phase of the therapy cannot be over-emphasized. It is one thing to be a catalyst in the deconstruction of clients' or families' mythology; it is another to provide them with the opportunity to revise their stories in such a way that these will be more in line with what they want. To omit the re-vision process is to leave the clients in a state of "psychological free fall." Alternately stated, it is to leave them outside of a story. As Patrick (1991) has pointed out, there is not much safety outside of a story; instead, there are only feelings of disconnection, lack of frame of reference, and uncertainty about where people belong and how they are to know. Without a sense of being part of a "shared story," people's lives seem to have little direction or meaning. Polkinghorne (1988) has stated this as follows:

> Narrative is a scheme by which humans give meaning to their experiences of temporality and personal actions. Narrative meaning functions to give form to the understanding of a purpose to life and to join everyday actions and events into episodic units. It provides a framework for understanding the past events of one's life and for planning future actions. It is the primary scheme by means of which human existence is rendered meaningful. (p. 11)

As therapists, we do not want to leave our clients outside of an old story, with no clues or help concerning how to be inside a new story based upon a description of their experience that is meaningful and accurate for them. For as Tappan and Brown (1989) have clearly stated, when people author their own stories, they clearly express their own moral perspective; they honor their own thinking, feeling, and doing with respect to what is right and wrong; they assume responsibility for their own moral actions; and they express their own sense of identity and authenticity. It follows that a meaningful therapy will help clients gain a sense of "being their own experts" via enabling them to author stories based upon their experiences, thoughts, and feelings. Furthermore, that such a therapy will help people address the central issues of their lives—that is, how they can live in a manner that, to a reasonable degree, gets them what they want and need. George Howard (1989) has eloquently made this point as follows:

> Science can tell us a good deal about how things function—this is (roughly) the domain of knowledge. Scientific psychology can tell us a good deal about how it is that people actually do function. But, for human beings, the question of how people ought to live their lives is also very important—this is (roughly) the domain of wisdom. Since science can tell us little (or nothing) about how we ought to live our lives, we begin to glimpse some of the roots of the scientist-practitioner problem in psychology, since psychotherapy frequently centers around questions of how one ought to lead his or her life. In A Story About George my reflections on "why I think, act, and feel the way I do" are of interest to me-as-a-scientist. But of even greater importance to me-as-a-person are questions about: what would make my life worth living; what values should permeate my relationships with others; what is the place of the spiritual in my life; and what are my proper responsibilities to my family, friends, profession, country, and the human race? For glimmerings of answers to such questions, one would be ill-advised to query science! Instead wisdom should be sought from the humanities, the arts, and enduring cultural institutions such as family, religion, and the schools, for knowledge is insufficient to give purpose to one's life. Purpose and meaning exist when one sees himself or herself as an actor in some larger story—be it a cultural tale, a religious narrative, a family saga, a political movement, and so forth. (p. 77)

We have become increasingly concerned that, to a large extent, our training has inadvertently predisposed us therapists to be much better at story deconstruction than at story re-vision. This is especially true of training that attempts to emulate the medical science model. In the extreme case, a therapist can even unwittingly become one more source that seeks to interpret a client's experience to her/him, rather than encouraging the client to become her/his own author. The therapist can take the client's experience from her/him, author what it means via a diagnosis and case notes, and by so doing suggest that the client cannot do that for herself/himself. In such instances, whether the therapist realizes it or not, he/she has sided with a view that "normalizes" certain ideas and practices representing the grand narratives of the culture, instead of being informed by a perspective that brings forth the dominant cultural specifications in order to "normalize" the right of persons to have their own separate accounts (Zimmerman & Dickerson, personal communication, 1993). A useful therapy, we suggest, is one that connects them to meaningful narratives compatible with their preferences, instead of separating and isolating people via placing them outside of "normal" stories and dramas. It is very easy to separate and exclude people via diagnostic systems suggesting that they do not belong in a "normal" story. It has been hard for us to understand, however, how such a procedure is useful in helping clients feel connected to meaningful contexts that they can use in authoring their own stories. It is our hope that this chapter will at least partially supply readers with tools that will aid them in inviting their clients to become their own authors, to trust their own experiences, and to find a voice to give language and form to the accounts that are thereby generated.

OUR DEFINITION OF FAMILY THERAPY

Since we view the process of therapy as basically a process of story deconstruction, re-vision, and connecting, we should clarify what we mean when we use the phrase "family therapy" before introducing a case example and describing specific reauthoring tools. Our view is quite different from the traditional notions that family therapy means having as many members of the family in each session as are willing to attend, and that a family therapist usually does not (if ever) see individuals. Our conceptualization of family therapy refers to a way of thinking rather than a particular type of treatment. Individuals compose families, families compose cultures and sociopolitical systems, and cultures and political systems compose countries. There are individual stories and story interactions at each of these levels, as we have previously pointed out. Individual stories are important in relation to shared or colliding stories, and shared or colliding stories are important to individual stories. We think in these terms, whether we are seeing an individual or a group of individuals (e.g., a family or a business). From such a perspective, "family therapy" can be conceptualized as a frame of reference that emphasizes the interconnectedness of all stories, and that is informed by this notion as we attempt to interact with clients in a useful way. "Family therapy" can thus be done with individuals, families, businesses, governments, and potentially even countries. It can be done with one person, dyads, triads, or any other numerical unit that seems useful. Some of our most successful work has been done with individuals whose family members were unwilling or unable to attend therapy. These cases were informed by a narrative family therapy frame of reference, however, and much of the therapeutic outcome was probably attributable to the relationship changes the clients began to initiate in their families. From our perspective, such work is family therapy.

CASE BACKGROUND

To provide a context for the therapeutic ideas that invite clients to become the authors of their own stories, we share in this chapter a case history in which these ideas were used. (Brief excerpts from various other case histories are used as well.) The case involved a female in her late 20s whom we will call Cindy. When Cindy requested therapy, she was enrolled in a graduate program and was in the process of working through a divorce, which had occurred a year previously. She explained her reason for coming to therapy as "wanting to get rid of some baggage from the past so that I can get on with my life." As Cindy described her situation, it seemed to the therapist that there had been a struggle going on for some time between an old story that had certain rules and specifications, and a potential New Story that had recently begun to emerge and could not be totally silenced. The old story had maintained quite an oppressive grip on her, via the notion that she would be rejected by her family if she changed too much. This had induced her to experiment in "responsible rebellion" from the family rules, in the hope that her parents and siblings would accept her and change their story about her. The result, however, was their inevitable nonacceptance of this "deviant behavior," and the tendency to create the rejection she so wished to avoid. Examples of her responsible rebellion were getting out of a marriage that she felt was very impoverishing for her; staying in school for too long (even if it was to get a graduate degree); and beginning to want to talk about and process the family's unspoken rules and regulations with her parents. At the time the therapy began, she was very much under the influence of anger and resentment toward her parents, which served to reify the family's story about her still further.

Cindy was also caught up in a repeating pattern in which she would declare her independence from the family, followed by contacting her parents in times of difficulty. These contacts usually resulted in their offering advice she did not want (treating her like a child), and Cindy's reiterating her declaration of independence. This would invite the family to feel rejected and misunderstood, and to cast her once again in the role of a rebellious, irresponsible child. Interactions of this sort influenced Cindy to attempt to prove that she was a responsible adult via cooperating with a perfectionistic lifestyle. This took the form of setting standards for herself that were impossible to achieve, always having more responsibilities than she could manage in a given period of time, and experiencing large amounts of pressure as a result. This effort to gain her parents' approval proved as futile as the others, and instead resulted in a deepening belief on their part in the old story. This repeated pattern, plus its recent escalation, had prompted her to come in for therapy in an attempt to re-vision her story. Her recent divorce, which was not compatible with perfectionism at all, seemed to add fuel to her desire to change, as it continued to be a source of confusion and guilt in her life. These patterns were discovered in the early sessions, which focused on the telling and deconstruction of her story.

TOOLS FOR INVITING CLIENTS
TO BECOME AUTHORS

1. Keeping Careful Track of Larger Themes That Can Inform New Stories

In keeping with the notion that the old story is largely shaped and informed by the narratives and meanings of others, especially those that would be considered large dominant themes, it follows that such themes will also be helpful in story re-vision. People's sense of being part of a shared story is connected to the feeling that they exist within some story larger than themselves. Mair (1988) has asserted: "We inhabit the great stories of our culture. We live through stories. We are lived by the stories of our race and place. It is this enveloping and constituting function of stories that is especially important to understand more fully" (p. 127). Howard (1991) has made much the same point as follows: "The young learn to tell the dominant stories of their cultural group—be those stories scientific, civic, moral, mathematical, religious, historical, racial, or political in nature" (p. 190). Accordingly, one of the most helpful things a therapist can do is to make note of larger themes and stories that clients can use to inform their re-vision process.

Information about dominant themes that can be used in the re-authoring process is potentially available from the very first moment of therapeutic contact. The therapist listens with an ear that is sensitized to hear such information. There will usually be many hints (if not actual statements) about the nature of these dominant themes during the early stages of therapy, when the client's old story is being told. Examples of such themes are religious affiliations, racial or ethnic ties, gender orientation, professional identity, and family tradition and history. If these themes are important in the old story, there is no need to assume that they must be totally abandoned or labeled as bad or ineffective in the new version. Rather, they need only be reinterpreted through being based on the client's experiences rather than the experiences and stories of others. For example, if the spouses in a particular family have been dominated by culturally stereotypical gender messages in their old story, it is quite meaningful to learn that the wife has been reading some feminist literature of late. This new version of what it means to be female may serve as the larger context to which she can refer in her new story. Simply deconstructing her old story will leave her outside of a story about gender; it is more helpful to identify new gender accounts that the wife will be comfortable sharing. Of course, a similar process can be conducted with the husband as well. New versions and meanings of such themes as these can be juxtaposed with old ones in such a way that restraints, distinctions, and differences can be rendered quite clear. In this way the clients still have stories with which they can identify, rather than finding themselves outside of an old story with no clue of how it can be reorganized or re-visioned.

In Cindy's case, it was not difficult to locate several dominant themes that could be used to inform her new story. These surfaced repeatedly in the course of the interviews. All that was required of the therapist was to listen attentively and make note of them as they appeared. When the time came to begin the re-vision process, several of these proved useful.

1. Cindy often mentioned how important being a good teacher was to her. She was serving as a graduate assistant at her university during the therapy, and her primary motivation for pursuing a graduate education was her wish to teach. It was obvious that she had strong feelings about this area and was committed to becoming as proficient a teacher as possible. It was interesting to note that the specifications about what it meant to be a good teacher that served to inform her came from a source other than her family, and were characterized by a very different view of the world.

2. Another dominant theme that emerged was the larger cultural story of what it meant to be female. The new cultural version of that story, as represented by feminism, was a very different interpretation of gender meaning than Cindy had been exposed to in her family. This new story of what it meant to be a woman had already partially captured her attention, thus presenting itself as a potential frame of reference for a re-visioned version of gender role.

3. Being well versed in literature, Cindy was also interested in the meaning of being human—the process of becoming a good person who contributes to society and the planet. This was a very large and somewhat general dominant story, but one that was important to her. Whatever new story she authored, it seemed sure that guidelines from this area would inform it to some degree.

4. The three previous examples were already in existence prior to the therapy. Another theme developed during the course of the therapy as a result of the dialogues between Cindy and the therapist. It involved Cindy's being invited by the therapist to ''tell your story with your own voice, based on your own experiences.'' This seemed to be very useful to Cindy, and she was intrigued about the implications of basing her story on her own interpretations of events, rather than on interpretations coming from others. This notion also served as an organizing principle for her new story.

2. Externalizing the Old/Problem Story and the Feelings and Thoughts It Uses

Over the past few years, the family therapy literature has seen an increasing number of authors espousing the "externalization" of client problems (White, 1984, 1986, 1988–1989; Epston, 1986; Menses & Durrant, 1986; Stewart & Nordrick, 1989; Tomm, 1989; Zimmerman, 1992). According to these authors, a therapy that "encourages persons to objectify, and at times to personify, the problems they experience as oppressive" (White, 1988–1989, p. 3) is more useful than therapies supporting the old definitions that clients bring to therapy with them. This view is based upon the assumption that clients' definition and understanding (interpretation) of their problems are often instrumental in supporting their continuing existence and power in their lives. Alternately stated, the survival story and the view of the world it habitually promotes suggest that a client continue to use certain solution behaviors that may have worked in the past, even if they have outlived their usefulness in his/her current life situation. As the client attempts repeatedly and unsuccessfully to apply old solution behaviors to the current situation, he/she is invited to feel more and more inept and powerless. We have found it very useful to offer a redefinition of the problem that invites people to construct new interpretations, and thereby to open space for re-visioned behaviors and solutions. The externalizing of a client's story, and the feelings and thoughts it supports, can serve as a very effective means of accomplishing such a redefinition. Toward this end, we often employ an "externalizing language" from the very onset of therapeutic contact with our clients.

Problem externalization involves talking about *problems* as problems rather than *people* as problems. Although this seems quite a simple notion, it is in direct contrast to the dominant "mental health story," which pathologizes people via placing their problems inside of them. There is a very powerful difference between describing a female client who has experienced a long history of being physically abused as a child as having a "self-defeating personality disorder," and suggesting that she has been highly influenced by a "male-dominated lifestyle." In the first instance, the problem has been located inside her in that vague, multiply defined area called "personality." In the second, it has been located in the familial and sociocultural context and definitions supported by the notion of patriarchy. In a self-defeating personality story, the client not only is held accountable for her abuse but is held at fault for it as well; in the externalized version, accountability is asked of the sociopolitical system, which has failed to require that men be more responsible in the expression of domination and violence. Patriarchy is a very powerful grand narrative, and an integral part of that story involves blaming victims for what has happened to them. When mental health professionals fall prey to that story, they run the risk of unwittingly supporting problem definitions that render their clients powerless rather than powerful. We have found externalizing the old story and its accompanying problems a very useful tool in the deconstruction process, as well as in story re-vision. We agree with White (1988–1989) concerning the outcomes of the externalizing process:

1. It decreases conflict between people over who is responsible for the problem.
2. It reduces the sense of failure people have in response to not having solved the problem.
3. It unites people against the problem rather than against each other.
4. It opens the way for people to reclaim their lives from problems.
5. It liberates people to view the problem in new ways.

From our conceptualization, we would add that it also is useful in enabling people to view the stories they brought with them out of childhood and adolescence in a more detached and curious way, to feel less responsible for these stories, and to talk about them as interpretations that may have been useful at the time. It seems to give them a certain distance (story deconstruction), which is useful in inviting them to consider a process of story re-vision, as well as giving them permission to do so. Externalizations change the title of a client's story from the Popeye-like title of "I Am the Way I Am" to one that can be summarized as "I Am the Way I've Been Influenced to Be." As Zimmerman (1992) has pointed out, the process of problem externalization is much more than a therapeutic "technique"; rather, it is a political view offering a perspective that stands in sharp contrast to the dominant cultural notion, which creates categories of abnormality via a "normalizing judgment." Zimmerman and Dickerson (in press) have summarized this nicely:

When one externalizes specifications in this way, one opens space for people's own preferred descriptions. One does not replace cultural specifications with therapeutic truths and solutions. To usurp systems of expert power (cultural, therapeutic), one begins to work in systems of personal power. From this perspective, self-actualization becomes the ultimate conformity, as it requires obedience to dominant and scientifically determined truths. Rebellion against these dominant cultural specifications allows people to begin to be influenced more by their own ideas/ideals of how they should be.

In Cindy's case, several externalizations were employed. The most effective seemed to be a very straightforward externalization of the old story, as well as the influence of perfectionism in maintaining the old story's existence. Examples of this process are provided in the end-of-chapter appendix; readers are also referred to Michael White's previously referenced publications for a more in-depth treatment of this topic.

3. Identifying and Becoming Alert to the Strategies Problem Stories Use to Stay Strong

Old stories and problem stories can be usefully viewed as having certain strategies, ploys, and contexts that they use to restrain change. Most often the client will be unaware of such restraints, in that they will not have been spoken or identified. White (1986) has suggested that such restraints are largely unconscious and take the form of "the network of presuppositions, premises, and expectations that make up the family members' map of the world and that establish rules for the selection of information about perceived objects or events" (p. 85). As such, these restraints are largely automatic and seem to be "just the way things are." In other words, the power that the problem story and its accompanying specifications wield is largely invisible or "unstoried." Examples of such unseen power strategies have been articulated by Zimmerman and Dickerson (in press) as follows: "(1) isolation from others, eliminating the comparison of experiences; (2) evaluation along harsh specifications as compared to normative classifications, with surveillance used to monitor the comparison; (3) rejection of personal experience through disbelief created by another, with the resulting dominance of another's experience over one's own." The purpose of the process outlined in this section is to render such restraints visible—to reveal them as extensions of a problem story and the interpretations it habitually supports. We have found this a useful process both in deconstructing the old story and in providing space for story re-visions.

Most often, it seems, clients describe these restraints in terms of feelings. Among those most frequently mentioned are fear, guilt, self-depreciation, perfectionism, and anger. Many readers have undoubtedly experienced such feelings themselves, and can relate to the restraining and impoverishing effects that they invite. Actively exploring these feelings often opens space for change via relaxing the constraints and constrictions they evoke. Since feelings are often accompanied by thoughts, this exploration also invites the clients to identify what such feelings are telling them (in other words, it externalizes them), as well as the particular types of contexts in which this occurs. As pointed out, such thoughts have quite often not been examined or admitted (or, if admitted, not processed).

It has been helpful to us to view this particular process as ''going on spy missions'' against the old story. This has proven a useful way of interacting with children (especially males). This analogy seems to sum up the intent of the assignment: gathering all possible information on the thoughts, feelings, and contexts that the old story/problem story uses to remain strong—and doing so in an orderly and systematic way. The process is much the same as scouting an opposing sports team with the intent of discovering how it manages to win so often. Instead, the scouting report is on the old story and the strategies and ploys it has used to authors client's life. This information can be used to devise countering strategies that the client can utilize to re-vision the story.

It seems important to note, however, that a metaphor of competing, opposing, and conflicting may not work well with all clients. It often fits a male version of the world better than a female one (although this is not always the case). It is important to match the metaphor to the client. If a client does not relate well to this ''battle'' metaphor, it can be altered somewhat. One way this can be accomplished is to ask the client to explore the ''gifts and lessons'' the old story has to offer, instead of coming up with counterstrategies to '''combat'' the Old story. After the lessons that need learning have been identified, the therapy can center around what a re-visioned story will look like once this has happened.

In Cindy's case, this procedure was used in a manner that invited her to stay aware of the types of contexts and interactions used by the old story to remain powerful in her life. Because she was a student, it was suggested that she "study and research" such instances to discover how they helped maintain the old story's existence. She proved quite adept at this, and in the process identified some of the behaviors she was cooperating with that helped things stay the same. For instance, she recognized that when she contacted her parents in times of difficulty, they were invited to treat her as if she needed help. She decided that in her re-visioned story, this pattern needed to be broken via relying on herself more as an expert on her own problems.

4. Exploring Specifications of Personhood

Michael White (1983, 1986, 1988a) has postulated that "specifications of personhood" are among the major restraints that can keep individuals and families stuck in stories they would like to re-vision. These specifications can be thought of as a "text" to which people refer in order to determine how they are to behave as individuals or as family members. To extend this analogy even further, such specifications can be viewed as the plot of a novel that has been primarily contrived by authors or forces external to the character (client) in question. External sources such as family, church, and culture form the frames of reference that people tend to use to define their "selfdom." Such specifications can be liberating and helpful, but when they are attached to an old story that has largely outlived its usefulness, they tend to become part of the restraining influences that keep impoverishing lifestyles strong. Stereotypical gender specifications serve as an excellent example. Individually, strict adherence to such roles can be quite restraining, and clients can find themselves so severely under the control of such notions that their lives are quite literally not their own. When this is the case, they can live, think, and act according to a gender story that has become problematic for them. Interactionally, when partners enter into relationships that are initially based upon such external standards, and when one of them subsequently begins to change, drastic relational difficulties can result. Resentment, anger, confusion, and distrust are common presenting symptoms in such cases.

When such specifications become evident while we listen to

clients' stories, we have sometimes found it useful to ask the clients to explore the specifications more closely and in a somewhat formal way. The details of this procedure have been outlined in a previous publication (Doan, 1991). The general procedure is presented here, using Cindy's case as an example.

During the early interviews, the therapist asked Cindy questions designed to explore what outside influences might be pertinent in relation to the problem she was experiencing. This led to an increased understanding that many of her specifications of personhood had been authored by someone other than herself. At this point she expressed a willingness to explore such specifications more closely. It was decided that it would be helpful if she actually wrote the "specifications-of-personhood text" that she had unwittingly believed and followed. This took the form of writing each of these specifications on separate 3 × 5 cards. When the cards were reviewed, they were found to contain items about what it meant to be female, what it meant to be a daughter, and what it meant to have a relationship with a man. Once these cards were generated (she managed to come up with some 70–80 of them over the next 3–4 weeks!), Cindy "sorted" them according to those that were helpful and those that were not. The guideline used for this sorting was for Cindy to focus on one specification at a time, read it aloud to herself, ask herself who wrote it, and process how it invited her to feel and think. If it invited liberating, expanding, and positive thoughts and feelings, she was to keep it. If on the other hand, it seemed to evoke constraining, impoverishing, and negative thoughts and feelings, she was to separate it into a stack that would be processed further at a later time. The results of her work at this assignment produced three stacks of cards: (1) those she was sure she wanted to keep, (2) those she was sure she wanted to discard, and (3) those that were placed in an "undecided" category.

This exercise is useful for some clients in providing them with a distinction between the kind of information that has informed the old story, and the type that can inform the re-visioned one. It is yet another way of providing distinctive differences between various interpretations and meanings, which can promote clients' viewing their lives as one version of a sequence of events rather than as reality itself.

It also has the potential to liberate portions of the old story and its rules via bringing specifications to light that were or are unspeakable in the family. An example of this in Cindy's case was the specification that women were to manipulate men by using sex, and feel superior to them because they could. Both she and her sister (who attended one interview) agreed that this specification was accurate in their family, but that it could never be mentioned or talked about; if it ever was, it would be denied. This had led both sisters to form the conclusion that if a female liked sex, she would be less likely to use it as a controlling mechanism, and that this was unacceptable within the family. That is, to be sexual was to risk rejection and lack of approval. They both agreed that their mother was the author of this specification, and that their father was ignorant of it (or at least pretended to be).

5. Developing the Rules of the Old Story versus the Rules of the New Story

Another means of providing a distinction between the old story/ problem story and the new story/re-visioned story, is to render the "rules" the old story has relied on visible, and to juxtapose them with rules that will support a new interpretation of the person's life. This is a somewhat different process from that outlined above concerning specifications of personhood, in that the rules of old lifestyles are more general in tone, whereas specifications are very specific. The intent of such a process is similar to those previously outlined: to change that which has been implicit into something explicit—in other words, to examine something that has been habitual and automatic in such a manner that it can be seen and reinterpreted. It is informed by Gregory Bateson's (1980) notion that differences and distinctions that lead to change invariably involve at least "two somethings," and Michael White's (1991) suggestion that the naming of a "counterplot" or an alternate story is often quite helpful in promoting story re-visions. We have found that comparing the rules that have helped maintain the existence of the old story with ones that would allow the person the opportunity to author a newer version is often a useful way of creating space for a client to begin living according to his/her preferences.

In Cindy's case, the interviewing process resulted in her deciding that perfectionism was the main source of keeping the old story strong. Identifying and examining some of the "rules of a perfectionistic lifestyle" seemed to be quite helpful for her. The development of such rules can be a natural extension of the externalizing process previously outlined. Examples of therapist–client dialogues, and rules that have been generated by such discussions, can be found in the appendix to this chapter. Readers are also referred to a previous publication (Doan & Clifton, 1990) for a more detailed look at this process.

6. Telling-of-Multiple-Stories Exercise/Experiment

In keeping with the notion previously presented—that clients are stuck in one interpretation of their lives, which is primarily based upon paying attention to certain events at the exclusion of others—we have found it useful to have clients practice alternate interpretations via re-visioning certain life events, as well as attending to some of those previously overlooked or censured. Put simply, this involves practice in the telling of various stories about the same sequence of events. This concept can be well illustrated by a case example in which a very concerned and scared mother showed up for her first therapy session with a copy of an abnormal psychology textbook under her arm and pronounced, ''I have found my son in here!'' She had read the book and had been able to pick certain behaviors from her 4-year-old son's life in support of a story that could have been titled ''On the Road to an Avoidant Personality.'' Among these behaviors were an intense fear of strangers, a tendency to spend lots of time alone, several imaginary friends, and resorting to prenatal posturing in times of stress and fear.

While listening to the mother explain about how she had constructed such a story concerning her child, the therapist began wondering whether some alternate interpretation would account for such behavior. Several options seemed worthy of exploration. When asked whether she would be interested in another story about her son, the mother enthusiastically indicated that she would. A series of questions was then presented about a story entitled ''Shy, Sensitive, and Intelligent.'' The mother was intrigued at the implications of this direction, and remembered that she had been extremely shy as a child herself. In fact, she recalled engaging in many of the same behaviors that were causing her to be so alarmed about her child. The session concluded with an exploration of which story she preferred to inform her interactions with the child. She decided to experiment with parenting on the basis of the "Shy, Sensitive, and Intelligent" story, and to report back on her progress. Several weeks later, a phone call revealed that the mother was now convinced that the shy hypothesis was probably correct, and that steps were being taken to invite her son to escape its influences more often. She indicated that she felt much more comfortable parenting from this stance, and that the influence of her fear had lessened a great deal.

This case led to an exploration of this process with other clients and situations, and although it is not a miracle cure, it has consistently proven useful. In its purest form, it is framed as a suggestion or experiment for clients to try between therapy sessions. It is suggested that when the clients are confronted with troublesome situations (anger, fear, self-depreciation, perfectionism, etc.), they tell themselves at least three stories about what is happening. The first story is to be the one that trouble would be most likely to tell (i.e., the one that would be supported by the old story and its interpretation of things). The others are to be alternate explanations, meanings, and interpretations of the same set of events, or interpretations including events that have been left out of the first story. In the case cited above, the mother had omitted her childhood shyness from the "On the Road to an Avoidant Personality" story. When this was added to the picture, a different interpretation was invited. This exercise constitutes actual practice in story re-vision. It concludes with the clients' asking themselves which version best fits who they want to be, or which version they feel will be the most useful.

It is also possible to involve family dyads, triads, or other groupings in this telling of multiple stories. A case example of this process was provided by parents who had just received word from their son's school that a recent battery of tests had shown the boy to be learning-disabled. The parents were both caught up in a story about this event that could accurately be entitled "Focusing on the Worst-Case Scenario." They cooperated with the multiple-stories process, and picked a different version that could be entitled "Maximizing Opportunity and Limiting Trouble." This process can be facilitated via questioning in the therapy session. Examples of such questions are provided in the appendix of this chapter.

Another interesting distinction that we have used in this regard employs punctuation as a metaphor: We ask clients to wonder about the difference between living life on the basis of a period as opposed to a question mark. Periods tend to invite a frame of reference that uses a language of givens, facts, and unchanging certainties, whereas question marks invite a language of wonderings, ponderings, and multiple possibilities. The multiple-stories exercise provides clients with an experience in living life from a questioning stance.

7. Rituals of Story Re-Vision and Reauthoring

Our ideas in regard to rituals have been primarily informed by the work of Evan Imber-Black (1988), who has been wonderfully inventive in using them to promote and maintain change in individuals and systems. These ideas have also been stimulated by Joseph Campbell (Campbell & Abadie, 1984), Sam Keen (1991; Keen & Fox, 1989), and Robert Bly (1991), and their notion that change occurs quite often when people are in what they call "ritual space."

Rituals occur in all cultures. The human species has the tendency to ritualize major life transitions and changes. In short, rituals play an integral and important part in the "human story"; to omit them from our thinking when conducting narrative family therapy would seem a major oversight. This has been summarized quite well by Imber-Black (personal communication, 1985): She asserts that family activities that we normally take for granted (meals, bedtimes, parties, etc.) are often highly ritualized procedures, just as holidays, life transitions, and religious ceremonies are. To put this in terms of our work, rituals can be conceptualized as the way the "speaking animal" marks the transitions and changes that occur in individual, family, and cultural stories. According to White and Epston (1989), rituals can be usefully employed in the conceptualization of individual and family crisis as "relating to some aspect of a transition or rite of passage in the person's life" (p. 17). This is very similar to our metaphor of symptoms as a "wake-up call"—a call inviting persons or families to reinterpret their lives in a way that will be less painful and troublesome for them. From this perspective, rituals can be seen as involving three phases (vanGennep, 1960, Turner, 1969):

1. The separation phase, which is marked by a departure from some status, story, or identity that has outlived its usefulness in the person's or system's life.
2. The liminal or "betwixt and between" phase, characterized

by confusion and uncertainty, but also by a heightened expectation about the future.
3. The reincorporation phase, signified by a re-visioned story or status that specifies new responsibilities for those involved.

This view invites therapists and clients to entertain questions about what a re-visioned story might be inviting the clients to separate from; what clues they might attend to about how their story might be re-visioned; when and how this new story might emerge; and how this whole process might be ritualized to render it clearer and more meaningful.

In Cindy's case, the notion that she needed to separate herself from some of the specifications identified on her 3 × 5 cards suggested a possible "rite of passage" to mark the beginning of this transition. In response to questioning about how she would like to begin this separation process, she indicated that it would be helpful to burn up the specifications she would like to leave behind. The session concluded with the suggestion that she think about this more and let the therapist know when she would like to do this, where she would like for it to occur, and whom she would like to be in attendance. She later reported her decision to burn the cards at the therapy office, with her sister in attendance as a witness and validator of the process. The therapist suggested that some other witnesses might be helpful, and wondered whether she would mind if other therapists observed the session from behind a mirror. Cindy indicated her acceptance of this suggestion, and also agreed that videotaping the session would be acceptable. The therapist also wondered whether Cindy might want to bring a container for the ashes of the cards, in order that she might keep them as a symbol and reminder of her journey.

The burning of the specification cards was conducted as planned, with both the therapist and Cindy making metaphorical comments during its course. These included noticing that some specifications seemed more reluctant to leave than others, and that even in the act of leaving a couple of them still tried to "burn" her. Her sister proved a wonderful addition to the ritual by agreeing that most of the specifications were accurate, and that she had been influenced by most of them as well. The group of therapist observers were also enlisted as a reflecting team (Andersen, 1987; Miller & Lax, 1988), which gave Cindy the opportunity to listen to their reactions and wonderings. (Please refer to Chapter 4 for a more detailed account of the reflecting team's purpose and activity.) Cindy indicated that she had decided to place the vase for the ashes on a special shelf in her home, where it could serve as a daily reminder of her new story. She was also provided with a copy of the videotape of the session.

It is well to keep in mind that although rituals can serve an important part of the process of change, they do not necessarily constitute change in and of themselves. Miracles should not be expected by either clients or therapists. However, if viewed as powerful invitations for reinterpreting and re-visioning, rituals can serve a very important function in narrative family therapy.

8. Pretending "As If" Assignments

The concept of pretending can be simply stated as "Fake it till you make it." We have found it a useful procedure with some types of clients. It is primarily used after the old story/problem story has been deconstructed, and clients have begun to identify and imagine some aspects of the re-visioned story they would like to author; however, it can also be used to juxtapose the old story and the new story for the clients to compare. For example, a client can be asked to imagine what sort of character she/he would be in the new story. On the basis of this description, the therapist can wonder about what would happen if the client pretended to be that character and behaved accordingly. The new pretended role can be alternated with the old pretended role (the one the client has been playing) for the client to compare. This can be done according to an "odd day, even day" ritual format in which the client plays the old role on Monday, Wednesday, and Friday, and plays the new role on Tuesday, Thursday, and Saturday. On Sunday the client chooses which of these fits better and plays that character, or else chooses some other version that might be better still.

A case in which this procedure was employed involved a middle-aged male who had been depressed for some 17 years. He had been to several therapists during this time without success. During the early sessions it became clear that his mother's opinion of him played an important role in the existence of depression, and that he viewed his mother as not approving of him at all. The therapist wondered whether this man had been pretending that everyone viewed him in the same way his mother did. He responded that this was entirely possible. A pretending "as if" experiment was suggested, in which the client would actively pretend for 1 week that everyone he came in contact with would view and respond to him in the same manner as his mother, followed by 1 week of pretending that others would view and respond to him in an entirely different way from his mother. The client tried the exercise and reported that he realized he had been living most of his life based on the assumption that everyone was like his mother. This opened the door for a re-visioned account in which this was not the informing principle.

9. Noticing and Documenting Re-Visioning That Has Already Occurred

As previously pointed out, every story is a form of censorship in that it is based upon paying attention to certain events at the exclusion of others, as well as applying particular meanings to the events thus selected rather than other possible meanings. It is quite easy for people to get so caught up in the story being told, along with the performances of meaning that it invites, that they are unable to attend to events and meanings that offer different accounts of the situation. We often encounter this in cases involving adolescents, their parents, and their teachers. Such cases are characterized by the adults' having storied the adolescents in such a way that behaviors that are *not* problematic or irresponsible are somehow overlooked or discounted. For example, an adolescent who begins lying to his/her parents is often storied as no longer being trustworthy, in spite of the fact that most of the time the adolescent tells the truth. The lying instances are attended to so strongly that they negate long periods of truthfulness. In fact, it is not uncommon to find that one occurrence of lying can negate or erase 10 to 20 instances of telling the truth! The adolescent becomes known as a liar—a title that disregards all information contradicting this story. This often invites the adolescent to take a "what's the use" attitude, to lose any motivation to change, and to take on a "career" of lying.

David Epston (1989b) has suggested that a human life is too rich and too varied to be encapsulated by only one story; such an effort will always censor out certain events and aspects of the person's life.

We concur with this notion, and would add that therapists are just as apt (if not more so) to tell only one story about people as anyone else. It is very easy for a therapist to fall prey to the problem story, to reify it, and to give it authenticity via labeling it and treating it. Furthermore, we suggest that this is just the sort of process encouraged by traditional thinking and training. Most of us have been trained (at least at some point) to focus upon what is wrong with people and families, to assign that "wrongness" some sort of diagnostic label, and to "know" what the people involved should do to correct the situation. The therapist who consistently sees "resistance" in her/his clients is engaging in a process that can be viewed as very similar to the parent–adolescent "liar story" outlined above. Rather than being trained to look for behaviors that are exceptions to the problem story, we have been traditionally trained to be experts to focus even more stringently on evidence supporting its existence. Epston (1989b) asserts that most stories contained in counseling center files are detective stories in which clues for pathology are searched for and investigated, and that the vast majority of such case notes read like a tragedy. In this section, we offer our readers an invitation to story their clients' lives in a manner that is quite different from this dominant pathologizing version.

It is our opinion that in most cases clients involved will have already begun a re-visioning of their lives. Often, the fact that they have come in for therapy is evidence that such a process has begun, and that they are seeking to extend it further. In most cases, however, they will be unaware that this is so, and will not be giving themselves credit for the movement they have already made. This will usually be characteristic of significant others in their lives as well. Michael White (1988a) has expressed very similar notions in his discussion of people with long-standing problems. He has asserted that because of the specifications of personhood and relationships to which people have been subjected, they will be blind to any information that contradicts a problem-saturated description of themselves and their relationships, and they will be predisposed to attend to and select out "facts" that support these long-standing definitions of themselves and others. Such "mythologies" are formed during a time in which the persons involved have no way of knowing how competent and strong they will become as they mature. As long as such long-standing definitions remain dominant, their acquired strengths and competencies will tend to remain unseen in spite of evidence to the contrary. It is important, if the process of re-vision is to continue and expand, that these competencies and strengths become accessible to the clients. It is highly advantageous for the therapist to be an expert at listening with "a constructive ear" so that this process can be facilitated (Lipchik, 1988; Lipchik & de Shazer, 1986).

The process of listening for evidence that a client has already initiated least a partial re-vision begins by having more interest in what is strong, adaptive, and resourceful about the client than in what is wrong, broken, or pathological (White, 1989). When the therapist is truly more interested in storying the client in such a manner, it is amazing how much evidence for such an account will be discovered in therapeutic conversations. For example, a male client with a long history of drug abuse came in with the story that he had fallen back under the influence of prescription opiates for 3 months. He, along with the significant others in his life, had storied this occurrence as a "relapse," and all were highly inclined to discount the gains he had made against this type of lifestyle. The therapist, instead of being primarily interested in "facts" that would support this story, instead expressed an interest in why the client had only used drugs for 3 months and had then quit on his own. As this story was recounted, the client begin to tell how the drug usage had been much less than on previous occasions, how he had not used alcohol at all this time, and how he had managed the affairs in his life much more responsibly than on the previous occasions. This established a very different tone for the session, and led to the opportunity for the therapist to juxtapose the old "drug-dominated" story with the more recent "drug-influenced" story. The client was quite intrigued with this line of thinking, and left more determined to try to continue lessening the power of the old story in his life. What could have become an instance of reifying failure and framing the client as unsuccessful was converted into an opportunity for renewed efforts that could be based upon the evidence of his progress, in spite of a counterattack by the old story.

We are extremely interested in any and all indications of story re-vision, no matter how small they might seem. Our thinking in this regard has been highly influenced by Michael White (1986, 1988a, 1988–1989; White & Epston, 1989) and Steve de Shazer (1982, 1985). Such instances of story re-vision can be thought of as unique outcomes, which are in contrast to the problem-saturated story a client has been living. Since these are apt to be overlooked or discounted, part of the reauthoring process involves rendering them noticeable to the client. These unique outcomes can be used to invite the client to consider an optional view of herself/himself upon which a re-vision can be based. However, this can only occur if the client is able to distinguish the differences as meaningful and noteworthy. Within narrative therapy, this is accomplished by inviting the client to story these events in a unique way. White (1988b) has succinctly described one way in which this can be done within the session. This process is outlined in the appendix at the end of this chapter, and interested readers are referred to White (1988b) for further information.

10. Asking Clients the "Miracle Question"

A process similar to that outlined above has been developed by Steve de Shazer (1988) and Insoo Kim Berg (1992) in the form of a "miracle question." We have found this to be most useful in inviting clients to imagine that change has already occurred. The questions is as follows: "Suppose that when you go to sleep tonight, a miracle happens and the problems that brought you here today are solved. But since you are asleep, you don't know that the miracle has happened until you wake up tomorrow. What will be different that will tell you that a miracle has happened?" Such a question invites a client not only to imagine that change has happened, but to give a detailed account of how the next day will be different as a result. It is recommended that the therapist obtain the re-visioned description in as much behavioral detail as possible, starting with the very moment the client awakens in the morning. Such a description will contain very small changes—changes that are quite possible for the client to achieve. It is also recommended that this account be about how the client will change as an individual, and *not* about how others will change. The reader is referred to the end-of-chapter appendix for an example of this process.

11. Uniting Individuals' Stories with the Stories of Others

As has been previously outlined, each of us is the central character in our story. While we are busy at that role, we expect and hope that others will play adequate supporting parts in our story. They of course, are hoping for and expecting the same thing from us. So each of us, simultaneously, is playing the central character in our own drama, expecting help from our supporting cast, and being asked to play a supporting role to the central roles of others. When such roles and expectations mesh, all is well, but when they collide and began to exist in opposition to each other, severe relational issues quickly develop. Such a collision of stories is often what brings families in for therapy.

In such cases, we have found it useful to have each member consider the above-described issues in a somewhat formal, thoughtful manner. This involves asking each member of the family to respond to the following questions:

1. What is my story, where did it come from, who wrote it, and what role is important for me to play?
2. What supporting roles do I need the other members of my family to play in my story?
3. What supporting roles am I willing to play in the stories of others in my family?

This exercise has proven useful in a variety of ways, since its completion yields information on a variety of fronts. First, it asks that each individual family member know his/her own story well enough to be able to relate it to the others. This is not a trivial task. Often people have not considered their relationships in such a systematic way. If individuals are unable to share their stories, it is very difficult for others to know what supporting roles to play. Second, it invites people to relate, in specific behavioral terms, what sorts of support they need and expect from others. This can be instructive both for the person doing the relating and for the listeners. It can render explicit that which has previously been implicit. Third, and perhaps most importantly, it invites all family members to actively consider the stories of the others, and to operationalize the ways in which they are willing to respond to them.

If this exercise is completed, it generally yields information that can be used for quite some time in therapy sessions. If the family members do not cooperate with the intervention, a session can be conducted that explores their understanding of not doing the exercise, and what they think it would mean if they did explore such issues. This can lead to a deconstruction of the story that has re-

strained them from sharing such information. Readers are referred
to a previous publication (Parry, 1990) for more information on this
intervention.

12. Family "Talking-Stick" Sessions

In keeping with the theme of finding the voice to author one's own
story, and the importance of stories that connect people rather than
keep them apart, we have found it useful to use family storytelling
sessions to accomplish both of these ends. As we have already pointed
out, families that come in for therapy have a tendency to be
"problem-focused." This invites them to develop accounts of themselves that stress the ways in which their various individual stories
are in collision, and to be unaware of accounts that would emphasize ways in which they are connected. Pursell (personal communication, 1992) has found that many of the families he has encountered
in a drug and alcohol treatment program were keeping information
concerning the ways they were connected a "secret," while the ways
in which they were in conflict were recognized by all concerned. He
has reported quite good results in asking the members of such families to "share the connections they have been keeping secret."

Pursell's approach is very similar to our intervention of asking
families to share family stories by using a "talking stick," which is
passed from member to member (Parry, 1991b). This is done after
a therapeutic discussion is held concerning the role thus far played
by storytelling and sharing within the family. The family members
are then asked to schedule a time and place about 1 week in the future when they will gather for the sole purpose of sharing family stories. The therapist asks that all members place these meetings on
a first-priority basis, and instructs the members to use the week to
think of some favorite family happenings. Old photos, family albums,
or any other kind of memorabilia can be used to aid in remembering or in telling these stories. To facilitate the meetings, the family
is instructed to obtain a talking stick; this can be a makeshift at first,
but perhaps one can be carved or specially selected as a family project
later. The person holding the stick is the only one with permission
to talk; everyone else is to listen. The stories told in this phase of
the exercise are to be happy stories, stories that are not told at someone else's expense. They are to include memories of good times that
the family members shared. When one person finishes a story, the

stick is passed to the next person, and the process continues. We suggest that these sessions be scheduled to last not more than 1 hour or less than 20 minutes.

A second type of story-sharing session can be included if deemed necessary, for the purpose of sharing experiences in which there is an embittering and excluding clash of perspectives, and blame has assumed dominance. The talking stick is employed in the manner outlined above, with each story being told as experienced by the person herself/himself, and excluding what the others did or did not do. Those without the talking stick are not to comment, but are instructed to listen carefully. When each person has related how she/he experienced the events, the story-sharing session ends with each member expressing appreciation and caring for the others. The talking stick is placed in an agreed-upon place of significance where it can be readily found for the next meeting, which is to be held not less than 1 week and not more than 2 weeks hence.

It might be good to note that this intervention is not the exclusive property of ''families in trouble''; it can also be used as a preventive measure in families that are quite content. Doan's own family has such meetings from time to time, and Doan has noted that the children call these meetings as often as the parents. It seems that they intuitively recognize the healing power of shared stories and request them as needed!

13. Family Stories That Control
versus Stories That Allow Personal Control

Elizabeth Stone (1988) has written a wonderful book on family stories and how they shape our lives. She examines the stories that were passed down in her own family, as well as those of some 100 others. The impact of this work in our own lives, together with that of George Howard's (1989) work, has stimulated us to view the family stories of the clients we see as rich sources of information for both us and them. Not only do such stories carry information about the familial traditions and meaning constructions of the particular people involved; they also can be very useful in both the deconstruction and re-vision phases of therapy. As family tales told in the therapeutic environment, they help reveal the major sources of authorship that were influential in penning the scripts, which the family members have been invited to accept as "just the way things are." In the telling, it often becomes obvious that the beginnings of the beliefs, actions, and expectations with which each family member identifies significantly predate the members' individual stories. This can have the liberating effect of inviting people to view their lives as "processes," rather than as "things" fixed in space and time. It can also encourage them to wonder about how these particular stories, and the meanings attached to them, were selected while others were left out. The telling of such stories opens the window through which the mythology (stories held in common) of a particular family can be viewed, examined, and challenged.

Metaphorically, this process may be similar to reading the opening chapters of a novel, after which the reader can become the author of subsequent sections rather than just continuing to be a player in an old, already written account. It seems that people need to hear and examine these stories, even if only as a prologue, in order to author their own. Unexamined stories remain not only unchanged, but powerful. They do so as major carriers of narrative meaning concerning the implications of belonging to a particular family in terms of gender, religion, ethnicity, race, and so forth. Until such stories are told, they are seldom examined; until they are examined, they are seldom viewed as optional; until viewed as optional, they are seldom changed. As stated by George Howard (1989),

> . . . at its core, human thought is storytelling. Some stories allow people to have greater control over their lives, whereas other stories picture people as pawns to other powerful forces in their lives. In believing that one cannot self-determine, a person actually brings about (or creates) the reality that he or she cannot self-determine . . . some stories are simply more hopeful than others. And certain people, like therapists, ministers, and so forth, are trained to discriminate "winner" from "loser" stories, and to help the person retell (or reconceptualize) the story in a way that is more hopeful. (p. 140)

Optionality implies choice, and choice implies having at least "two somethings" to compare. As long as only one something exists, no awareness of choice or optionality is possible. Some family stories imply that there is only one correct way to be; such stories render optionality "taboo" in that particular family. Elizabeth Stone (1988) has made this point quite nicely:

The family is our first culture, and, like all cultures, it wants to make known its norms and mores. It does so through daily life, but it also does so through family stories which underscore, in a way invariably clear to its members, the essentials, like the unspoken and unadmitted policy on marriage or illness. Or suicide. Or who the family saints and sinners are, or how much anger can be expressed and by whom.

Like all cultures, one of the family's first jobs is to persuade its members that they're special, more wonderful than the neighboring barbarians. The persuasion consists of stories showing family members demonstrating admirable traits, which it claims are family traits. Attention to the stories' actual truth is never the family's most compelling consideration. Encouraging belief is. The family's survival depends on the shared sensibility of its members. (p. 7)

This "shared sensibility" implies that everyone in the family should have this view, and anyone not doing so runs the risk of censure and rejection. Thus, instead of inviting optionality, diversity, and role exploration, many families invite conformity, singularity, and unquestioning loyalty via the spoken and unspoken stories they share. The message is conveyed that there is only "one story," which is the one ordained by the family. Other stories are not considered; if they are, it is with suspicion and harsh judgment.

Given this line of thinking, we have found it useful to invite our clients not only to share their family stories, but to categorize them by dividing them into one of two groups: those influencing people to be controlled by others' versions of them, and those suggesting that people can be the authors of their own lives. This exercise creates the "two somethings" necessary for optionality, as well as inviting clients to analyze the message or intent of family stories and narratives. They can then engage in a much more informed discussion concerning which stories they feel are useful for them in their process of re-vision, and which they would like either to alter or to leave behind.

14. Parenting to Protect versus Parenting to Prepare

The approach described in this section is included as a "metaphor" or a "prototype" that can be used with many other distinctions and areas of concern. Space does not allow us to include a comprehensive treatment of all the story distinctions and juxtaposings we use in the re-vision process. We hope that this story about parenting to protect versus parenting to prepare will invite readers to create their own story titles that their clients can use to clarify their lives.

Once upon a time, there was a therapist who had encountered a steady stream of family cases in which the parents seemed to be having great difficulty in altering their parenting strategies and stances as their children grew older. It seemed to this therapist that such parents were stuck in a story about what it meant to be good parents—a story that had no room in it for a re-vision appropriate for children as they reached adolescence, and the accompanying "attack of the great hormone monster." The regular outcome of this scenario was that the parents would apply more and more rules and control, and the adolescents would respond with more and more rule breaking as statements of individuality. That is, the parents would treat the adolescents more like irresponsible children, and the adolescents would respond with behavior that would invite the parents to do this even more. Of course, the adolescents' version of this was that they were not going to be treated as if they were still children, and that the parents needed to wake up and realize this was so.

Perhaps this is a familiar story to some readers. Perhaps readers have found themselves, like the therapist in this story, wondering how such a cycle can be interrupted so the family can move into a more useful sequence of interactions. It was in the middle of just such a family therapy story that the therapist found himself involved in the following dialogue:

THERAPIST: Let me see if I've got this right. Currently, your story about what it means to be a good parent is primarily informed by the notion that your job is to protect your child—to see that nothing really bad even has a chance to happen to her?

MOM: Yes, I think that's accurate. That is what good parents do, isn't it? No parent would let something bad happen to their child if they could prevent it.

THERAPIST (to *Dad*): Do you agree with your wife? Does this sort of thinking influence the way you parent as well?

DAD: Yeah, I suppose it does. I guess I'd say it a little bit differently, though. I think we've been overprotective. Up until she was 16, she didn't have to take care of anything . . . we did it all for her. I think that's been a problem in a way.

THERAPIST: How has it been a problem? And (*to Mom*) do you agree with him?

DAD: It has been a problem in that she's had no training in how to do things for herself.

MOM: I probably don't think it's been as much of a problem as he does, but I would agree we probably did too much for her.

THERAPIST: So it sounds like that both of you agree that you've done a great job of parenting to protect, but you wish you'd done a little better job of parenting to prepare?

DAD: Yes, that's accurate for me. (*Mom nods her head in agreement*)

THERAPIST: So would it be fair to say that early on in your daughter's life, you very successfully and appropriately parented in such a way that she would be safe and protected . . . and that it worked for both you and her during that time? But now, the story of parenting to protect seems to have somewhat outlived its usefulness, and both you and your daughter are wondering if it isn't time to move on to a new parenting story?

MOM: Well, that might be true. She certainly doesn't seem to want as much protection any more! But it's really hard to do, so many bad things can happen to them out there.

THERAPIST: Yes, the world we live in today really requires a very well-prepared person, doesn't it? How important would it be to both of you that your daughter be prepared to face it?

DAD: Obviously, it would be very important. I don't think we've done a very good job at that.

THERAPIST: Perhaps it wasn't time to until now? I wonder if your daughter would have been ready much earlier?

MOM: I don't think she would have. It's hard for me to think she's ready now.

THERAPIST: Would she be ready to begin this process? I wonder if that's what some of her rule-breaking behavior has been trying to say.

DAD: It's time for her to be ready. In only a couple of years we're expecting her to go off to college!

THERAPIST: It sounds like maybe you are both ready to try experimenting with parenting to prepare your daughter instead of parenting to protect . . . even though fear will make it hard for you to do. Is this something you would be interested in?

MOM: I'd be interested, but it will be hard to do. We might need some help.

We have subsequently found this distinction, which spontaneously arose in this session, to be quite useful in cases where parents are struggling with the most useful posture in relationship to their children. It seems to effectively create the "two somethings" from which to offer clients glimpses of alternate stories. The comparison of a narrative entitled "Parenting to Protect" with one called "Parenting to Prepare" not only provides clarity, but suggests that successful and caring parenting can be conducted from more than one stance. We suggest that such distinctions render the process of revision much easier, and we use them as often as possible.

15. Emphasizing Conflicting Stories Rather Than Conflicting People

If the experience of most family therapists reading this book matches that of our own, significant portions of their caseloads have been composed of families in which conflict has entered the system during puberty and the adolescent developmental period. These cases have always been problematic for us, because it seems that the stakes are usually quite high for both the parents and the adolescents, and as a result each side is firmly entrenched in a particular viewpoint. Recently we have been experimenting with a new approach when confronted by such cases.

This process was stimulated by the work of George Howard (1991), in which he suggests that many of the conflictual problems between parents and adolescents can be usefully conceptualized as cross-cultural struggles:

> Many of the classic struggles between parents and their children in adolescence and early adulthood come about as children espouse the values and beliefs of their subjective subgroup that conflict with the beliefs and values of the parents' subjective culture. Stated in terms

of this article, struggles for independence by adolescents and young adults represent cross-cultural struggles as much as do misunderstandings and conflicts among members of different religions, races, nationalities, and the like. The stories advocated by the subjective cultures of adolescents often clash with the storied perspectives held near and dear by their parents. (p. 192)

The notion that *stories* are conflicting or colliding, rather than *people*, has been very liberating for us. It suggests a therapy that seeks to address the manner in which the stories are conflicting, rather than the way in which people are in conflict. Parent–adolescent conflict seems an excellent example to illustrate this process, although this is certainly not the only type of case in which this sort of thinking can be employed. It is possible to invite those on any two sides in an existing conflict to entertain the notion that their respective stories or interpretations are in collision, rather than the people themselves.

This can be illustrated via Figure 3.1, a "reciprocal-invitations map" drawn from the types of interactions that can be typically observed in parent–adolescent struggles. As the cycle shown in Figure 3.1 continues, each episode of nonconformity may get "more serious," with the result that the parents are invited to create even stricter rules. By the time therapists see such families, it is not uncommon for the adolescents' nonconforming behavior to have reached pro-

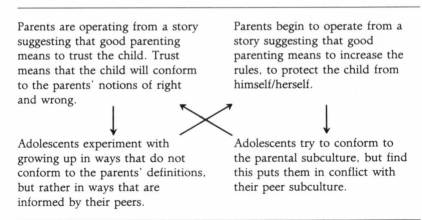

Parents are operating from a story suggesting that good parenting means to trust the child. Trust means that the child will conform to the parents' notions of right and wrong.

Parents begin to operate from a story suggesting that good parenting means to increase the rules, to protect the child from himself/herself.

Adolescents experiment with growing up in ways that do not conform to the parents' definitions, but rather in ways that are informed by their peers.

Adolescents try to conform to the parental subculture, but find this puts them in conflict with their peer subculture.

FIGURE 3.1. Example of reciprocal-invitations map drawn from parent–adolescent interactions.

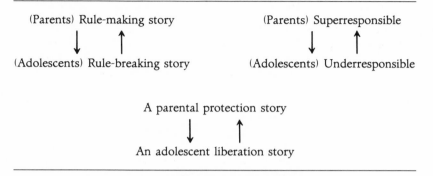

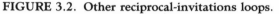

FIGURE 3.2. Other reciprocal-invitations loops.

portions that are causing them problems with the school and the legal system, as well as with their parents.

Other reciprocal-invitations loops that can be identified are illustrated in Figure 3.2. In such situations, mixed invitations and meanings usually abound. Parents send messages that imply ''Grow up, but I don't trust that you can''; adolescents send messages that can be summarized as ''Treat me as if I'm grown up, but continue to protect me if I mess up.'' Also, adolescents can find themselves being ''caught between two stories''—feeling unable to cooperate totally with the story of their parents' subgroup, and at the same time being censored for trying to share a story with their own subculture. While this is going on, parents can be involved in mourning the loss of a story for their children—a story that has been part of their dreams for a long time.

When such reciprocal-invitations patterns are encountered, we have been experimenting with sending the family members home with a prepared list of questions to consider prior to the second session. These questions are informed by the notion that it is useful in therapy to address the dominant stories or meaning domains (i.e., what it means culturally and familially to be ''good parents,'' and what it means to be ''good adolescents'' within the youth subculture) that are inadvertently supporting the continued existence of the problem. This work assumes that until space is provided for the alteration of the dominant stories informing people's behavior, change in behavior will be extremely unlikely. The handout given the family members is presented in Figure 3.3.

FIGURE 3.3. Handout on parents' and adolescents' stories.

Parenting is tough work. Being an adolescent is tough work, too. In fact, these may be two of the toughest jobs in the world! It is really little wonder that families can often fall under the influence of trouble and conflict when parents are trying as hard as they can to be true to a "parents' story," while adolescents are trying as hard as they can to adhere to an "adolescents' story." Parents' stories are very different from adolescents' stories, and are characterized by notions suggesting that parents must always protect their children no matter what they do; that they are ultimately responsible for what the children do or don't do; and that if the children are not successful, then it means the parents have failed as parents. Adolescents' stories tend to be made up of notions suggesting that their parents are too old ever to understand them; that their friends and what they think are just as important as their parents; that no matter what they do, their parents can't be pleased; and that their own job is to discover who they are rather than to become like their parents. It is very easy for stories such as these to collide. It is just as easy for those involved to take such collisions personally, rather than to see them as cross-cultural differences. Within such story interactions and collisions, fear can began to dominate, and can influence all parties involved to resort to very extreme behaviors in the search for solutions.

In an attempt to turn the tables on conflict and fear by examining the colliding stories upon which they depend, the following questions are suggested for your consideration. It is recommended that both parents and adolescents use these questions to review their own stories, so that the collision aspects of the stories can eventually be revised into ones that can be shared.

P = questions to be answered by parents
A = questions to be answered by adolescents

1P. How good is your son/daughter at getting you to side with the story that good parents are superprotective of their children's lives? What sorts of things does he/she do to accomplish this?

1A. How good are you at getting your parents to believe that they should be superprotective of your life? What sorts of things do you do to get your parents to believe they should be superprotective of you?

2P. How good are you at inviting your daughter/son to side with a story suggesting that adolescents aren't capable of assuming responsibility for their lives? How do you accomplish this?

2A. How good are you at getting your parents to cooperate with the story that they aren't good parents—that if they were, you would be more responsible? How do you manage this?

3P. How has it come to pass that you are caught up in a story suggesting that good parents have to work harder at their children's growing up than the children do? What are the "rules" in your parenting story supporting this notion?

3A. How has it happened that you are cooperating with a story that has you believing that it's your parents' job to work harder at your growing up than you are? Are you ready for your parents to start believing that you are willing to do your own work at growing up, or would it be too soon for you to handle this?

4P. What sort of pressures will make it hard for you to change your story about being superprotective of your adolescent?

4A. What sort of pressures will make it hard for you to take the responsibility for your own growing up?

5P. Which story would suit you best: to continue to side with the notion that you have no choice but to accept your daughter's/son's invitations to be superprotective of her/him, or to stand up to these invitations and invite your adolescent to be responsible for her/his own life?

5A. Which role would fit you best: to continue "growing down" and getting your parents to be even more protective of you, or to continue growing up and inviting them to let you be responsible for yourself?

6P. If you wanted to revise your story so that you could stand up to the invitations of superprotection, what are you currently doing that you would want to do even more of?

6A. If you wanted to revise your story so that you could stand up to the invitations of growing down, what are you currently doing that you would want to do even more of?

7P. If you parents got together on a regular basis to discuss your parenting story and the invitations it makes you to be superprotective of your son/daughter, do you think you would be able to help each other revise this story? Could the two of you devise an "escape plan" from this old story?

7A. If you took the time to think regularly about the invitations that growing down makes to you, do you think that you would be able to come up with ways to stand up to it? What sort of an "escape plan" could you come up with in order to insure that you grow up?

8P. What behaviors (if any) could your son/daughter engage in to show his/her individuality that would be acceptable to you? In what areas could your adolescent be different from you, and this would be OK?

8A. What behaviors that are different from the way your parents are could you use to express your own voice that would have the best chance of being accepted by them? If they accepted your individuality in these ways, would that make a difference in your relationship with them?

9P. In your definition, is good parenting synonymous with producing children who largely conform to your view of the world? Or is it to produce children who are independent and think for themselves?

9A. Do you view your job as an adolescent as forcing your parents to realize their view of the world is wrong by acting out and rebelling? Or is it to invite your parents to realize that you are capable of making your own decisions about who you want to be?

10P. If you viewed your daughter's/son's nonconforming behaviors as an experiment in individuality (which is based upon your adolescent's living in a very different world than you did at her/his age), rather than as rebellion against you, would that change anything?

(continued)

FIGURE 3.3. Continued

10A. If you viewed your parents' behavior as designed to prepare you for life away from home (based upon their view of the world), would you see them any differently than you do now? Are you ready for life away from home?

11P & A. If you began seeing the conflict in your family as a by-product of different views of the world, rather than as personal issues between people, would it invite you to do anything different?

12P. How much of your time and energy would you want to spend in parenting to protect versus parenting to prepare? Which would be most important—that your son/daughter be protected from the world or prepared for the world? How has your parenting been divided between these two in the past?

12A. Which would you want your parents to do more of—parenting to protect you or parenting to prepare you? Have you been inviting them to protect you more or prepare you more? If they were willing to parent to prepare, how would you be willing to respond?

The reactions of the family are processed in the next session, which is scheduled 2 or 3 weeks in the future. Although this intervention is certainly not a "miracle cure," we have found it useful in providing space for an ongoing discussion of the stories involved, and in creating of room for stories that can be shared.

We should note that therapists can select various questions from Figure 3.3, rather than requesting that family members answer all of them. Also, these certainly are not all the pertinent questions that can be generated, and we hope therapists will be stimulated to develop others that are relevant to specific families they are seeing.

16. Inviting Responsibility via Examining Intentionality

We are interested in discovering as many alternate ways of inviting clients to examine their stories as we can. We are particularly interested in methods that encourage both clients and therapists to understand the origin and the motivating forces behind the stories in question. Recently we have discovered an intriguing notion in the work of Gary Zukav (1989). He has suggested that people's intentions have a large influence on the various realities they can create as they interact with the world. He goes so far as to suggest that in every moment of consciousness there is an intentionality that interacts with the behaviors, and thus every action reflects some sort of intention or motivation. For example, if people intend to protect themselves from potential hurt at the hands of others, their behavior will be quite different than if their intention is to be open and trusting. From Zukav's point of view, the internal narratives that people construct are largely guided by their intentions. Most individuals, however, are not aware of their own intentions; or, if they are, they consistently hold other people responsible for them. Using Zukav's work as a platform, we have become quite interested in inviting our clients to explore their own intentionalities, as well as to own the responsibility for them.

As we have experimented with such an approach, we have become aware that therapists have intentions as well, and that an examination of therapists' intentions while they are in the process of interacting with clients is also a potentially very fruitful area of inquiry. Do the therapists intend to give advice to their clients, to tell them how to live, to coconstruct a reality with them, or merely to reflect what they have said? From this point of view, therapists' intentionality is every bit as important as the clients'.

In order to introduce such a concept into therapy or supervision, we have developed an intentionality worksheet, which is designed to introduce clients or supervisees to the process of exploring their own intentions. It is our hope that once people have had the experience of thinking in these terms, the stage will be set for further exploration via therapeutic questioning and dialogue. The worksheet we have developed is presented in Figure 3.4.

FIGURE 3.4. Intentionality worksheet.

The intent of this worksheet is to provide you with the experience of exploring your own intentions and motivations. By "intentions" we mean the constant process of deciding what the events in our lives mean, and how we are to respond to them. Every action therefore reflects an intention. This exercise will invite you to think about some experiences you have had, and the intentions that informed your behavior.

Following is a list of intentions that humans can have. It is not a comprehensive list, and you may feel free to add any others that may come to mind. Please read through the list quickly, and then turn to the second page to continue.

(continued)

FIGURE 3.4. Continued

1. To hide my feelings
2. To conceal my thoughts
3. To remain mysterious
4. To escape some situation
5. To be cautious
6. To protect myself
7. To attack someone
8. To expand the options
9. To enable someone
10. To experience happiness
11. To gain freedom
12. To have security
13. To dominate physically
14. To dominate psychologically
15. To convince someone
16. To humiliate someone
17. To strengthen someone
18. To protect someone
19. To grieve
20. To hurt someone
21. To help someone
22. To have the answers
23. To know for sure
24. To include someone
25. To allow differences
26. To be smarter than someone

27. To be deliberately curious
28. To explore new ideas
29. To withhold judgment
30. To cooperate with someone
31. To be an equal partner
32. To appear cool
33. To have my act together
34. To keep my options open
35. To keep growing
36. To take a one-down position
37. To be a victim
38. To be taken care of
39. To be the responsible one
40. To gain revenge
41. To give away responsibility
42. To make someone understand
43. To allow someone space
44. To seek attention
45. To pay attention
46. To make someone feel sorry
47. To know myself
48. To hide from myself
49. To ignore the situation
50. To follow the rules
51. _____ (any others)

Now that you have read through the list of various intentions, please use them to complete the exercise below. For each scenario suggested, select the three intentions *most like* how you felt at the time, and the three intentions *least like* how you felt. We have found it useful, as you remember the incident, to ask yourself first whether you felt comfortable or uncomfortable. Then decide which intentions guided your behavior.

1. Remember, as vividly as you can, an interaction that was *pleasant* with a significant other who was *not* a member of your biological family. List whom the interaction was with, and the intentions you selected, below.

Person _____

Three intentions most like   Three intentions least like

_____   _____

_____   _____

_____   _____

2. Remember an interaction you experienced as *pleasant* with a member of your biological family.

Person _____

Three intentions most like   Three intentions least like

_____   _____

_____   _____

_____   _____

3. Remember an interaction that was *unpleasant* with a significant other *not* in your biological family.

Person _____

Three intentions most like   Three intentions least like

_____   _____

_____   _____

_____   _____

4. Remember an interaction that you experienced as *unpleasant* with a member of your biological family.

Person _____

Three intentions most like   Three intentions least like

_____   _____

_____   _____

_____   _____

Read over the intentions you have selected very carefully. Construct a brief story about the person they describe. Tell the story in the third person, as if you were an observer of this person. Describe his/her character, motivations, and view of the world. How do this person's intentions differ in situations that are pleasant versus ones that are not? What intentions does he/she prefer? How much of the person's time is spent in intentions that are preferred versus those that are not? Limit the story to the space provided. [At this point, the rest of the page is left empty for the story the respondent generates.]

After the completion of the worksheet, which we often send home with clients, a therapist can process the results in a session. We have found this a very useful process with some clients; it invites them to be more aware of the parts they play as individuals in interactions that prior to this work have largely been "automatic." Examples of the types of therapeutic questions that can be employed are included in the end-of-chapter appendix.

CONCLUDING COMMENT

In writing this chapter, we have not intended to claim that it represents a comprehensive list of therapist–client tools and procedures for story re-visions. Our intent has been to present those that have proven the most useful in our work over the years. We hope that the ideas presented here will enable other therapists to expand this type of thinking into even more effective ways of empowering change in the "storytelling animal."

APPENDIX: THERAPEUTIC EXAMPLES

1. Keeping Careful Track of Larger Themes That Can Inform New Stories

Case Dialogue Example

The following case dialogue is offered as an example of the process of keeping track of larger themes. There are many ways in which this can be done; the important point is that the therapist needs to listen with an ear tuned to hear such information.

THERAPIST: It seems that in the old story you were taught to primarily use your professional identity to define and give meaning to yourself . . . that the story you brought into young adulthood maintained that you are what you do for a living. Does this match with your understanding and experience?

CLIENT: Yes, that has always seemed true for me. I've always placed a great deal of importance on my job. That has been the major part of my life for some 25 years.

THERAPIST: And this story served you very well for some time. In fact, until just the last few years you were quite successful professionally—and felt pretty content.

CLIENT: Yes, that seems accurate . . . except for the perfectionism thing, of always having to do things perfectly and putting lots of pressure on myself.

THERAPIST: Yeah, there was that, but up until a few years ago you wouldn't have described yourself as depressed . . . you hadn't tried to kill yourself?

CLIENT: Yes, I was certainly a lot happier than I've been the last few years, that's for sure.

THERAPIST: But then things started to happen that invited you to find other ways of defining yourself. You lost the job you'd had and loved for a long time. Not only did you lose it, but the way you lost it—because of another person's jealousy. This allowed depression to enter your life. That sort of got depression started.

CLIENT: Yes, that is pretty much the way it happened. I just couldn't adjust to it, especially when I couldn't find another job which was as good. I really got down during that time.

THERAPIST: That's when I first saw you, wasn't it—right after depression had convinced you to try and take your own life?

CLIENT: Yes.

THERAPIST: And things got better for a while. You fought back against depression and its buddy perfectionism, managed to get another job . . . were on your way to regaining control of your life. Is that accurate?

CLIENT: Yes, but it is hard for me to remember. I forget that I did pretty well for a while there.

THERAPIST: Yeah, bad times can sure make it easy to forget the good ones, can't they? But of course, having that stroke and brush with death didn't help, did it?

CLIENT: No, that was not what I needed. And losing my new job because of all the health problems didn't help either!

THERAPIST: That's for sure! And now . . . well, it seems that you are really being invited to come up with some other standard to judge yourself by. Were there any other things that were important in the old story—things that gave meaning to your life?

CLIENT: What do you mean?

THERAPIST: Other than your job, what else gave meaning to your life? Was it religion, what it means to be a male, family tradition . . . any of those?

CLIENT: No, not really. I've never been very religious, and the men's movement just doesn't interest me. The family tradition was all about work . . . that's all there was.

THERAPIST: How about what it means to be a good human being? Has that been important to you all along?

CLIENT: Well, yeah, sure. I've always tried to be a good person.

THERAPIST: Since the doctors are telling you to take it easy, since it appears you won't be able to work professionally like you did in the past, would it be time to replace the work story with one about being a good person?

CLIENT: Gosh, that would be hard. Being good involves working.

THERAPIST: Is that all it involves, or are there some other aspects to it?

CLIENT: There are other things as well.

THERAPIST: Like what?

CLIENT: Like being a good friend, being honest, being there for others. Things like that.

THERAPIST: I wonder how things would change for you if you let things like that define your worth instead of whether you can work? The work story seems to have sort of outlived its usefulness for you, although it was quite handy for a while. Is it time to use some other criteria for judging yourself?

CLIENT: Well, since I can't work much any more, I probably won't feel too good unless I am able to change that.

THERAPIST: Would you want to experiment with that for a while?

CLIENT: I can try.

This example represents a case where not many dominant themes had emerged (other than work!), and this had served as a major stumbling block in the client's progression. Hunting for and finding another dominant theme proved very useful in the client's story re-vision.

Some Useful Questions

• What sort of larger themes have been important in the old story: gender, race, family tradition, religion, others?

• Would you want the same themes that were in the old story to inform your new story? If so, would they need to be changed in any way? If not the same themes, what different ones would you use?

• Are there important people in your life with whom you feel comfortable sharing a story at the present time (or in the past)? What characterizes those shared stories that you would like to take with you as you continue your journey?

• What larger general themes have been the most enabling in your old story? Are there areas in the old story that you view as successful and liberating for you?

2. Externalizing the Old/Problem Story and the Feelings and Thoughts It Uses

We have found many uses for the concept of externalizing a client's problem, not the least of which has been the utility of this process in connection with traditional DSM-IV diagnostic categories. It is possible to externalize any and all of the DSM-IV labels, and in the process to reframe the meaning of such labels for both the client and the therapist. This is equally true of any feeling or emotion that a client may find problematic. This section provides general "rules" for externalizations, a sampling of externalizations we have found useful, and an example of therapeutic dialogue in which an externalization was called forth and used.

General Rules for Externalizations

1. Externalizations usually move from the general to the specific. The therapist begins with a general externalization (e.g., trouble), and moves to a more specific one as more is known about the client. However, this is not always the case; some clients prefer more generalized externalizations. The next rule helps clarify this decision.

2. Externalizations are best when they are phrased in the client's own language. We prefer externalizations that the client has created in response to therapeutic questions. For example:

THERAPIST: When depression is around, what does it feel like to you? What would you call it?

CLIENT: Well, it feels like an attack by an army of Blue Meanies.

3. The most powerful externalizations are those personifying the meanings that support certain symptomatic behaviors. For example, we have found that in cases of depression, the most useful externalization is often that of the standard of judgment that the client feels unable to meet. Feelings of worthlessness, helplessness, and hopelessness do not exist in a vacuum; rather, they exist in relation to some standard that the client feels unable to attain. Thus, an externalization of perfectionism (or some equally unachievable standard) often creates more positive change than externalizing the depression itself.

4. Externalizations may be connected to the childhood and adolescent survival story, so as to be placed in their historical context. This tends to invite the client to realize that she/he was highly influenced by external sources, rather than believing that "It's just me."

5. Interactional patterns that are occurring between people should not be overlooked as possible candidates for externalizations. Zimmerman and Dickerson (in press) have outlined such a procedure in their work with marital couples, in which they suggest externalizing the reciprocal invitations that are evidenced in the relationship. They offer an example that externalizes the husband's tendency to withdraw and be distant, and the wife's tendency to pursue and seek closeness. The therapist can then ask ques-

tions that call forth information about the influence of withdrawal on all concerned, as well as the influence of pursuing. Questions can also be asked about the influence of pain (or anxiety, or sadness—whatever feeling becomes evident in the couple's language), which may be the inevitable outcome of such interactions.

Examples of Useful Externalizations

Readers are referred to White, (1984, 1986, 1988–1989) for the basis of the following examples:

Depression: The influence of inertia; a helpless, hopeless lifestyle; a career of depression; the influence of unreachable standards or perfectionism.

Anxiety or fear: Tyranny of the fear monster; a worst-case scenario lifestyle; the influence of scary stories (this works well with panic attacks).

Anger: Tyranny of the anger monster; a hurt-in-disguise lifestyle; a career in being out of control; a "gunslinger" lifestyle (this is especially good with young fighting males); carrying on a tradition of family anger.

Anorexia/bulimia: A fear-of-food lifestyle; the domination of gender stereotypes; carrying on a family female tradition.

Encopresis/enuresis: "Sneaking poo/sneaky wee"; a baby lifestyle.

Irresponsibility: A little-girl/little-boy lifestyle; domination by the notion that "others should do it for me."

Hyperactivity: The "I've got to move" bug.

Theft: The influence of "sticky fingers."

Cyclothymia/bipolar disorder: A "yo-yo" lifestyle; an up-and-down lifestyle.

Alcoholism: An alcoholic lifestyle; a hiding-in-the-bottle career.

Adjustment disorder: The influence of major change; the influence of stress.

Physical/sexual abusiveness: A male-dominated lifestyle; the influence of male ownership; domination by patriarchy; habit of underresponsibility (Jenkins, 1990).

Codependence: A caring-too-much lifestyle; a career of self-erasure; a habit of living for others.

Sexual abuse: Having one's life storied by others; being robbed of one's own voice and experience; an at-fault, victim lifestyle; the influence of male domination.

Case Dialogue Example

THERAPIST: I understand that you are here because you've been visited by anger more often than you would like?

CLIENT: Yes, it seems I'm angry most of the time, and it has gotten a lot worse lately.

THERAPIST: So how much of the time would you say that anger is in charge of your life these days—25%, 50%?

CLIENT: Uhmm . . . gosh, that's hard to say. It is in charge a lot. It comes and goes and sort of depends on the situation. I guess around 50% of the time.

THERAPIST: When anger is in charge, when it manages to sort of take over, do you feel like a different person at those times?

CLIENT: Absolutely. I do and say things that are pretty bad. Things I wouldn't say when I'm not angry.

THERAPIST: Yeah, it's funny how anger works that way. When it is in charge, it convinces us to be totally different people. It can be pretty powerful that way.

CLIENT: Yeah, for sure! I can't seem to stop it.

THERAPIST: At those times, when anger manages to take over your life, how would you describe the way you are feeling? How would you describe the anger?

CLIENT: It's like an all-consuming rage, like I'm out of control.

THERAPIST: I wonder, at those times would you also be feeling hurt? How much of your anger would be hurt in disguise?

CLIENT: Uhmm . . . I've never thought of it that way . . . but now that I do, most of the time I'm feeling hurt. I feel hurt and I strike back. I feel hurt and I rage.

THERAPIST: So would it be fair to say that you have gotten in the habit of a rage-instead-of-hurt-lifestyle . . . that rage manages to use hurt in order to take you over and control you?

CLIENT: Yeah, that is pretty accurate, I guess, although I never thought of it that way.

THERAPIST: And how have you thought of it?

CLIENT: Well, it's just been me . . . an angry, out-of-control person who couldn't help it.

THERAPIST: So in the past, not only has rage been able to use hurt to take over, but it's also been able to convince you that it was in charge and there was nothing you could do about it?

CLIENT: Yes, again that is accurate . . . I've always been that way.

THERAPIST: So this hurt-as-rage lifestyle dates back a long time. Does it go all the way back to childhood?

CLIENT: Oh yeah, it goes all the way back.

THERAPIST: So you sort of brought this habit out of childhood with you. In what ways was it necessary for hurt as rage to exist back then? How did this help you survive?

CLIENT: I'm not sure what you mean.

THERAPIST: What I'm wondering is, what would have happened if you hadn't used anger instead of hurt as a child . . . is there any way that anger protected you back then?

CLIENT: Yeah, I guess so . . . nothing I ever did was good enough. I tried hard to be good enough . . . I still am trying, I guess.

THERAPIST: So the rage protected you from the hurt that you weren't going to be good enough—that nothing you did was going to get you the approval that you wanted? Sounds like maybe it kept you going, kept you from becoming depressed. If you had gone to your parents and told them you were hurt, that you needed more acceptance, what would have happened?

CLIENT: Nothing. They—especially my father—would have said that I had everything and should be grateful. He wouldn't have understood.

THERAPIST: So rather than show the hurt, you came to rely on rage instead of hurt, and it got you through?

CLIENT: Uhmm . . . perhaps I'll need to think about it.

THERAPIST: Of course, feel free to share those thoughts with me if you think it would be useful. But in any event, however rage got to be part of your early story, you are here because it seems to have outlived its usefulness . . . you'd like to change your story?

CLIENT: That's for sure. I need to change it. It's ruining my life.

3. Identifying and Becoming Alert to the Strategies Problem Stories Use to Stay Strong

Since the problem story gains its power during a time when the client has no idea how strong and capable she/he will later become, it can only stay in power if it can keep the client unaware of the strengths and resources she/he has developed in the process of growing up. It does so via a network of restraints that can be weakened if they can be revealed. We have thus found it useful to ask our clients to "do research," "go on scouting missions," or "spy on" the ways in which the problem story remains strong. To illustrate this process further, another example of therapeutic dialogue from the hurt-as-rage case (see above) is provided.

THERAPIST: Last time, we discussed you staying alert to the ways in which hurt as rage remains strong in your life. You indicated an interest in investigating this. Did you decide to do this over the last 2 weeks, or did something else seem more important?

CLIENT: I probably didn't stay as aware as I should have, but I did manage to identify a few.

THERAPIST: And what were those?

CLIENT: Well, rage really seems to be strong any time I am confronted by someone in authority—or maybe I should say confronted by someone I really want to respect me. In those situations, I have to be careful or rage will take over.

THERAPIST: Uhmm . . . it seems that those are situations in which what others think could be potentially hurtful. If they didn't respect you, that you would feel put down, or at least not appreciated for what you'd done.

CLIENT: Exactly. It's like if I don't get the credit that I think I'm due, then rage takes over immediately.

THERAPIST: So one strategy that hurt as rage uses to stay strong is to convince you that others must respect and appreciate what you do, and if they don't, then you have no choice but to cooperate with rage?

CLIENT: Yeah, that's accurate.

THERAPIST: Any others?

CLIENT: Oh yeah, there is a biggie—rush hour traffic! I can get almost crazy with rage during rush hour. It's like every other driver exists only to get in my way . . . like they do it on purpose.

THERAPIST: How about the traffic signals and lights? Are they put there by some idiot who knew it would inconvenience you?

CLIENT: Exactly!

THERAPIST: So hurt as rage convinces you to take lots of things personally—anything which inconveniences you. It stays strong that way.

CLIENT: Yeah, it sure seems to.

This process is continued until a representative list of strategies has been identified. Once this is done, the therapy focuses on ways in which the client can turn the tables on this old story, such that it better fits his/her life as an adult. In this instance, the client became very adept at not getting stuck in recursive conversations where he tried to convince others he was worthy of respect. Instead, he began to see such conversations as outdated vestiges of an old story that rage used to stay strong. Of course, as he began to try to convince others less, they became more invited to see him as a person they respected. As for the rush hour traffic, he devised strategies such as listening to his favorite soothing music, using the time to record notes on tape for his business, and sometimes choosing to avoid being on the road during peak traffic times. These re-visions put him more in charge of hurt as rage than it was of him.

4. Exploring Specifications of Personhood

Because we have gone into some detail concerning specifications of personhood in the main body of the chapter, only a few additional comments seem necessary here. Explorations of these specifications do not have to be produced in written form by a client. They can be elicited via questions within therapy sessions and recorded by the therapist; they can also be put on audiotape, or not recorded at all. The essence of this process is to render the specific rules that define the client's personhood visible for examination. This can be done in whatever manner seems most appropriate for the particular client(s) involved. Following are some examples of the types of questions used to elicit such specifications:

• How is your current story like or unlike that of your parents? How are the roles and expectations of the old story like or unlike that of your family of origin?

• If your parents were here right now, what role would they say you should play, given the circumstances you are in? What would be the specifications accompanying such a role?

• If you were to write down the specific rules of what it means to be a good person (or son, daughter, wife, husband, male, female, etc.), what would these be? Who would have authored most of them, you or someone else?

• What roles were you "hired" to play in your family of origin? What are the particular rules of this role—that is, what is required of you to maintain it?

• What sort of specifications would the old story rely on in order to remain strong?

5. Developing the Rules of the Old Story versus the Rules of the New Story

Case Dialogue Example

The following therapeutic conversation with Cindy (see text) illustrates the procedure of developing the old versus new rules. The distinction illustrated can be best summarized as juxtaposing "rules for staying the same" with "rules for changing." This process can create clear differences where there existed only one way of being previously.

THERAPIST: It sounds like you are beginning to know perfectionism pretty well—the invitations it makes to you—and that you've managed some escapes from its influences.

CLIENT: Yes, I believe that's true. I've been able to make much smaller lists of things I have to do. And even when the big lists sneak up on me, I manage to leave them somewhere during the day . . . just sort of lose them. (*Laughs*)

THERAPIST: Sounds like you are beginning to know perfectionism so well that you could even identify some of the rules it uses to control you?

CLIENT: Yes, I suppose I could.

THERAPIST: What are some?

CLIENT: You can never prepare too much.

THERAPIST: Never be too ready?

CLIENT: Yes.

THERAPIST: Any others?

CLIENT: You can never do enough, you have to keep pushing, pushing, pushing . . .

THERAPIST: Those sound very powerful and dominating. Are there others?

CLIENT: Perfectionism is an alone thing . . . no one can help you or it doesn't count. A Superwoman complex. But this time I broke the rule, I consulted someone else.

THERAPIST: You were somehow able to give that rule the slip this time. How did you manage it?

CLIENT: I decided that I could trust and share, that I had nothing to prove.

THERAPIST: Oh, is that another rule of perfectionism?

CLIENT: Yes. You always have to measure up to others.

THERAPIST: Does identifying perfectionism's rules seem helpful to you?

CLIENT: Yes, it makes it much more clear that it is destructive.

Some Useful Questions

Although it was not done on this occasion, these rules could have been juxtaposed with a new emerging set of rules in the client's life. Some questions that could have been asked in this regard are as follows:

• It sounds as if you have been developing some other rules to replace those that perfectionism has taught you—such as that it's OK to trust and share rather than compete. Did I hear you correctly?

• If you wanted to extend your ability to escape perfectionism's rules, what sort of competing rules would you need to come up with? Do you suppose there are rules for defeating perfectionism as well?

• Sounds like one of perfectionism's major rules has been the notion that you have to be Superwoman. How would you rewrite that rule so that it would be more useful to you?

• What sort of rule were you following when you decided to consult someone, rather than handle your life alone? How is this different from what perfectionism would have you do?

Another Case Dialogue Example

THERAPIST: So in the past guilt has visited you often?

CLIENT [female]: Yes, real regularly.

THERAPIST: What are some of the rules that guilt has used to stay strong in your life?

CLIENT: I might be wrong and they might be right.

THERAPIST: Who is "they"? Are "they" all males?

CLIENT: Yes, absolutely.

THERAPIST: So one rule is that the female voice is inferior to the male voice . . . that females should doubt their own experience.

CLIENT: Yes.

THERAPIST: Are there others?

CLIENT: Yes, another one is that I don't have the right to hurt anyone in the process of taking care of myself.

THERAPIST: So if you try and get your own needs met, and someone acts hurt because you do, your job is to quit and take care of them?

CLIENT: Yes, and of course that's usually males too.

THERAPIST: So all a male has to do is realize that if he acts hurt, you have to stop taking care of yourself. If he realizes that, he can get you to take care of him all the time.

CLIENT: Yeah, that's it in a nutshell! (*Laughs*)

THERAPIST: What sort of new rule would you want to replace that one with in your new story?

CLIENT: That I can care about people and be fair and kind to them, but I don't have to be totally responsible for their feelings.

THERAPIST: Yes, that would be very different, wouldn't it?

The Rules of Fear and Anger Lifestyles

The following rules (Doan & Clifton, 1990) have been generated in interactions with our clients over the past few years. We have found them useful in many instances, and sometimes give them to clients for their consideration—and additions!

- Fear and anger do not play fair. They will do anything to win.
- Fear and anger will "splash" on anyone who stays too close to them for too long.
- Fear and anger thrive when people try to pretend they don't exist; denial seems to be one of their favorite foods.
- Fear and anger also thrive on "quick fixes" or "miracle cures," but they are very allergic to small, progressive changes, and must leave if these persist.
- Fear and anger are tricksters, and love taking people unaware. As such, they are very sneaky much of the time.
- Fear and anger tend to lose strength if people can see them coming.
- Fear and anger usually start out small and grow very slowly. In this way, they can take control without people being aware; they can take their time and become habits.
- Fear and anger are only damaging when they are in control. They can even be quite helpful when people are in control of them.

• Fear and anger tend to make people allergic to successes and to pretend that these don't exist in their lives. The "eyes" are particularly susceptible to this allergy, rendering people "blind" to any successes that they might have.

• Anger often disguises itself as righteousness, while fear often masquerades as safety.

• Anger and fear use stereotyped gender roles to attack men and women.

6. Telling-of-Multiple-Stories Exercise/Experiment

Basic Steps

The multiple-stories procedure has been outlined in detail in the body of the chapter. The basic steps are reiterated here in the interest of simplicity:

1. When clients find that they are being lived by a story in which they are uncomfortable, they are to finish that story in complete detail to its worst possible outcome.

2. They are then to take the time to construct at least two more versions of the same events. These additional versions are to involve interpretations, meaning applications, and implications differing from those of the original story.

3. After at least three versions have been constructed, they are to ask themselves which version they feel would be the most useful for them and their families, which version best fits with the people they would like to be, and which would be most likely to lead to the story outcome that they desire.

4. After picking the version that best answers these questions, they are to experiment with living their lives "as if" this version were true.

Some Useful Questions

• I understand that the particular sequence of events in your life has invited you to tell me the story that you have. Would you be interested in an alternate account of the same events? What would you title the account you just gave me? Is there another title that would suggest a different interpretation?

• In my experience, when bad things happen in a person's life, it can be either an opportunity for growth or an invitation for trouble. I can certainly understand how you would be inclined to side with the notion that trouble is totally in charge, but is there another story? Is there a story about an opportunity for growth?

• It sounds as if, in your current story, parenting means protecting. Would you be interested in a story in which parenting would mean preparation? How would such a story be different from the current one?

7. Rituals of Story Re-Vision and Re-Authoring

Types of Rituals

There are many opportunities for the use of rituals in therapy. A complete treatment of this subject goes beyond the scope of this book. Here are a few of the many possible types of rituals and situations that observant therapists can use with their clients.

Religious holidays and ceremonies can be used ritualistically. The period of Lent in the Catholic Church is an excellent example. Family members can be invited to give something up for Lent that would tend to create a positive change in the system.

All types of holidays, birthdays, and traditional family observances can be used to generate therapeutic rituals. An excellent example of this can be found in the work of Evan Imber-Black (personal communication, 1985). She used the father's birthday in a blended family to help overcome the conflict being caused by the difficulty of merging the two biological sons of the father with the two biological daughters of the mother. Naturally, the parents were tending to defend their own children, and trouble and conflict had managed to use this to their advantage. The ritual involved asking the sons, as experts on their father, to help the mother and the daughters plan a surprise birthday party for him. This intervention managed to interrupt the existing coalitions in the family in such a way that new relationships and connections were invited.

Burning, burial, and freezing rituals can be used to help re-vision situations involving past events, secrets, conflicts, rules, or specifications that might need to be set aside or forgotten. These can take various forms, limited only by the imaginations of the therapist and client. The following examples are offered:

1. Family members or spouses can engage in ritual burying of a secret or a conflict that has managed to keep them from developing a satisfactory relationship. After the secret or conflict has been written on a piece of paper (or some item is selected to represent it), the burial is performed in an outdoor area quite a distance from the family home. The therapist, and any others the family members may wish to involve, serve as witnesses to the ritual. After the burial, the family is instructed that if in the future anyone brings up the secret or conflictual topic, the others have the right to tell her/him, to ''Go dig it up.'' The topic must then be dropped unless the

person is actually willing to return to the burial site and return with the buried item.

2. Freezing rituals can be used in a similar manner, with objects or notes frozen in bowls of water, which must then be thawed out before they can be discussed. This can be a nice ritual to mark the end of therapy, with some item symbolic of the change selected to be frozen. If any family member forgets and reverts to behaviors from the old story, the rest of the family can tell him/her, "Go thaw it out."

3. One use of burning rituals has been described in the text proper. This same sort of procedure can be employed with any object or conflict that clients are sure they want to leave behind.

Some Useful Questions for Determining Readiness

A word of caution is in order concerning all of the rituals suggested in this book. Timing is very important, and therapists should make sure that clients are really ready to move on to a new story. Questions concerning this readiness are suggested prior to engaging in any type of ritual to mark change. Some such questions are as follows:

• How would you know if it was time to discard certain aspects of the old story that you have indicated are impoverishing to you? What signs of readiness would you look for?

• If you tried to bury this secret before everyone was actually ready, what do you think would happen? Would it be important that all involved actually be ready to move on to a new story?

• I've found that guilt sometimes attacks people who try to change too fast. If you burned these specifications, do you think that guilt would be able to use this to attack you, or do you feel ready to take this step?

• What would you need to do to test your readiness to take this step? Would you need to test your readiness by putting the secret away for a week to see how it goes?

Some Useful Questions in Formulating Rituals

• If you wanted to take the step of getting rid of some of the specifications that you have identified as being impoverishing for you, how would you want to do that? This would seem like quite an important event to me. Would you want to mark it or punctuate it in any special way?

• If you wanted to leave this secret behind—sort of make sure that it isn't going to author your future story as a couple—can you think of a way that you could agree on doing that? Would you want to have a ceremony to mark its passing if you did?

• You have indicated that you'd like to burn up the specifications you want out of your life. Where would you like to do this? Would you want anyone special to witness the burning? How would you like for the burning ceremony to go?

8. Pretending "As If" Assignments

A pretending procedure can be used in almost any situation where a client has envisioned change but has not been able to "behave it." The following questions have proven helpful in this regard:

• If you could side with the vision of the new story that you have for yourself, what sort of things could you imagine yourself doing that are slightly different from what you are doing now? If you pretended that you could do those things, what do you think would happen?
• I understand your feeling when you say that if you joined with the new story, you would only feel you are "faking it." What I am wondering is whether you'd be faking it in the new story, or whether you've actually been faking it in the old story all this time? What if the old story has been a pretense? Which story would you rather "pretend at"—the old story or the new one?
• If you pretended, although you don't currently feel this way, that the positive things about you are just as valid as the negative ones, what difference would this make in your view of yourself?
• It seems in the old story that you have been pretending that you had your own voice, when it seems from your account of things that you've mostly been living according to others' versions of you. If you began pretending that you have a valid voice, what sort of things might you tell yourself to do?
• If you went home, set up your video camera, and acted out the character that you would like to be in your new story, what would the camera record you doing and being?

9. Noticing and Documenting Re-Visioning That Has Already Occurred

Michael White (1988b), in his article "The Process of Questioning: A Therapy of Literary Merit?", has described a most elegant way of noticing change that has already taken place and rendering it so distinct that the client and significant others cannot fail to see it. The reader is referred to this article for an in-depth treatment of this process; a summary of the four steps involved is also provided here.

The process involves the therapist's "calling forth" narrative accounts from the client, couple, or family via specific types of questions. The intent is to render the accounts so distinct that they are much less likely to be ignored or overlooked. Never underestimate the power of a good story!

Steps 1 and 2: Calling Forth Unique Outcomes and Accounts

Sample Questions to Elicit Unique Outcomes

- Can you recall an occasion when you could have given in to the old survival story but didn't?
- Can you think of a time when your relationship was facing adversity, and could have been overcome by trouble, when instead you rallied and warded off the problem?
- Can you think of an instance in which you managed, as a couple, to side with a new story rather than cooperate with the old problematic one?
- If you think carefully, can you remember an occasion when you managed to lessen the influence of trouble's old story, even though you didn't hold it off entirely?

Sample Questions to Elicit Unique Accounts

- How did you manage to step outside of the childhood survival story and fear on this occasion?
- Can you help me understand what sort of steps you took to be able to hold the old story at bay this time?
- Where do you think you got the idea for experimenting with a new story?
- What did you do in the past that prepared you for taking this step at this time?

Case Dialogue Example

CLIENT [female]: Life has no meaning any more. He left me for someone else, for a younger woman. I really don't care what happens. Nothing seems worth it.

THERAPIST: How is it that him leaving you, although I understand that would be very painful, means that life is not worth living? Could you help me with that?

CLIENT: I'm not getting any younger . . . I gave him some good years, years when I was very attractive. I'm not certain that I will be able to attract a man any more. It's all been a waste! I feel like such a fool!

THERAPIST: So time is running out, and you are under the influence of very scary stories about your future—stories which suggest that you are no longer attractive, and that you have used your time foolishly.

CLIENT: Yes, exactly. I don't even want to go to work any more. Nothing seems to matter.

[At this point the team with which the therapist was working called him out of the room. They were concerned that the depression was not only running the client, but running the session! After a brief visit with the team, the therapist returned.]

THERAPIST: The team is very curious about your story, and they are slightly confused. They wanted me to try and clarify some things for them. They couldn't help but notice that you are dressed very attractively today. One of the female members of the team said she didn't think she had ever seen makeup so tastefully applied. They were wondering, if this departed lover took everything with him—all the meaning in life—how is it that you managed to look so nice today? [Unique outcome.]

CLIENT: Well (*long pause*), I may have overstated it. He took a lot with him, but he didn't take everything!

THERAPIST: I see. He didn't take all of your pride, he hasn't managed to steal away your concern about your appearance?

CLIENT: No, not entirely.

THERAPIST: Are there other things he didn't take with him? Are there other ways in which you still care about yourself and life? [More unique outcomes.]

CLIENT: I suppose there are. I'm still working out regularly. I swim 5 days a week.

THERAPIST: Really! So he didn't take that with him either.

CLIENT: No.

THERAPIST: You also mentioned dreading going in for work. Have you been going in?

CLIENT: Of course, I haven't missed any work.

THERAPIST: So even though you have been sad and grieving for the loss of this relationship, you have still managed to continue working out, looking nice, and going to work. Is that correct?

CLIENT: Yes, but I have to do those things.

THERAPIST: Really? Who says so? I mean, you don't have to do any of them.

You could have given up on everything. How have you managed not to do that? [Unique account.]

CLIENT: Well, I still have some pride.

THERAPIST: So on the one hand, depression has tried to take over your life and convince you that it's not worth living—and on the other, it seems that you have a voice which has been very successful in keeping depression from gaining complete control of you. What do you think it means about you that you have been able to do this? What do you think it means to the team behind the mirror? [More unique accounts.]

CLIENT: Uhmm . . . well . . . I guess it means that I'm not quite as bad off as I could be. Maybe they think that there is some hope for me! (*Laughs*)

THERAPIST: Do you think that depression will be able to steal these things away from you, or are you determined to continue to take care of yourself by looking nice, working out, and going to work?

CLIENT: No, I don't think it will be able to get me to stop . . . it sure might make it hard, though.

THERAPIST: Yes, it could do that, but it sounds like you are determined not to let it gain more control than it has.

CLIENT: Yes, I suppose that's true.

Steps 3 and 4: Calling Forth
Unique Redescriptions and Possibilities

It is one thing for a client to engage in thoughts and behaviors that are unique in relation to the old story; it is another for such events to become note-worthy enough to form the basis of the client's new story. In our opinion, most of the clients with whom therapists come in contact already have evidence in their lives of alternate stories to which they are not attending (i.e., or which they are unaware). It seems, however, that the majority of the time these "solution-saturated" thoughts and behaviors are not being used to inform their stories about themselves. Instead, they are primarily "performing meaning" consistent with the portions of their lives that would lead them to believe that they are somehow deficient. In this section we will focus on techniques that invite clients to attend to aspects of themselves indicating that they are resourceful and adequate, and to give such characteristics more credence in the process of self-storying. As clients began to attend to different aspects of themselves and different events from their experiential pasts, and to apply different meanings to the events so selected, they are quite literally engaging in the process of re-vision. This is an extremely important aspect of the narrative therapy process, as the following statement by Michael White (1991) indicates:

The idea that it is the meaning which persons attribute to their experience that is constitutive of the persons' lives has encouraged social scientists to explore the nature of the frames that facilitate the interpretation of experience. Many of these social scientists have proposed that it is the narrative or story that provides the primary frame for this interpretation, for the activity of meaning making; that it is through the narratives that persons have about their own lives and the lives of others that they make sense of their experience. Not only do these stories determine the meaning that persons give to experience, it is argued, but these stories also largely determine which aspects of experience persons select out for expression. And, as well, inasmuch as action is prefigured on meaning making, these stories determine real effects in terms of shaping of persons' lives.

This perspective should not be confused with that which proposes that stories function as a reflection of life or as a mirror for life. Instead, the narrative metaphor proposes that persons live their lives by stories—that these stories are shaping of life, and that they have real, not imagined, effects—and that these stories provide the structure of life. (pp. 27–28)

Thus, the narrative analogy suggests that for human change to occur, the stories that structure and shape people's lives—in other words, the "meanings they are making"—must undergo some sort of re-vision. We hope that the following ideas will be useful to other therapists in helping clients entertain alternate meanings and aspects of their experience upon which to base their stories about themselves, others, and the world.

There at least two important aspects to this process: inviting clients to story themselves differently in their imagination and conversation, and inviting clients to experiment with behaving in ways that are consistent with this newly imagined view of themselves. As Coale (1992) has succinctly pointed out,

. . . while human systems are meaning systems and meaning is created linguistically, it does not logically follow that conversation (one evidence of linguistic understanding) is *the* route to a change in meaning. Change in meaning can occur through experience and behavior, symbolic and nonverbal communication, as well as through conversation. (p. 14)

In other words, new thinking can lead to new behaviors, as well as the reverse. In our view, therapists are responsible for inviting clients to do both: to re-vision themselves, and then to act on this re-visioned view. We use the conversational atmosphere of the therapy session to call forth new accounts and meanings from our clients, and rely upon suggestions and assignments that the clients implement between sessions to provide them with the experience of living their new stories, Steps 1 and 2 (unique outcomes and accounts) invite the clients to consider alternate events upon which to base their self-views. Steps 3 and 4 invite them to consider new meanings about themselves (unique redescriptions), as well as to imagine what behaviors might result from such a re-vision (unique possibilities). Thus, the first two steps are concerned with obtaining new accounts from clients, while steps 3 and 4 invite the clients to construct new meanings about themselves, as well as to imagine future behaviors that are implied by these alternate points of view. Examples of this process are provided below.

Sample Questions to Elicit Unique Redescriptions

• What does this victory over the old story tell you about yourself that would be important for you to know?

• What does this new story about Jane/John tell you about her/him that you somehow had not known before?

• How do you think this new account has changed others' view of you? How might their stories about you have changed?

• Do you think that this new information has changed how the team members think about you? If so, what new ideas do you imagine it has invited them to have?

• What do you think this tells others about you that they can appreciate?

• What does this re-visioned account tell you about your relationship that is pleasing for you to know?

Sample Questions to Elicit Unique Possibilities

• What difference do you think knowing that you managed to be your own author will make in your future steps?

• What new possibilities do you think have become available in the relationship with your parents (children, husband, wife, etc.) as a result of this new information?

• Now that I know this about you, what possibilities would you imagine I must see for you?

• Since you find this new story very liberating, in what ways would you want to side with it even more?

• If you were to identify with this alternate information about yourself, what do you think you will find yourself doing next?

• How will the attraction to this new story affect your view of yourself in the future?

Case Dialogue Example

THERAPIST: So you had several occasions over the past couple of weeks when you could have fallen prey to anger, but instead you walked away and decided it wasn't worth it. Have I got the story right?

CLIENT [middle-aged male]: Yeah, that's about it. Somehow I managed not to try and convince the other person of anything . . . and I also didn't take the fact that they disagreed with me so personally.

THERAPIST: Gosh, what a different story than when you first came in! It's pretty amazing, really. Did being able to do this feel good to you?

CLIENT: Oh yeah. It felt like I was in control.

THERAPIST: So you managed to handle a potentially conflictual situation in a very different way from the old story. I'm wondering, what do you think this means about you that you were able to do this [step 3]?

CLIENT: I'm not sure I follow you.

THERAPIST: Well, the person in your old story would have blown up, would have let anger run the show—but you didn't. Can you describe this new person for me?

CLIENT: Uhmm . . . it is different. I thought differently than before. I sort of saw Anger trying to take me over, and decided not to cooperate.

THERAPIST: I see. It means that you can now see anger, and make up your own mind, rather than just automatically letting it hold sway. It means you can think differently. Is that correct?

CLIENT: Yes, that's the way it happened. I really hadn't thought about it until you asked . . . but yeah, that's the way I remember it.

THERAPIST: How does it feel to know this about yourself, to know that you can perceive and think about a situation like this differently—a way that's not under anger's control?

CLIENT: It feels really good . . . it feels like I'm finally growing up!

THERAPIST: So would that be something else it means, that you acted in an adult fashion?

CLIENT: Yes, it's much more adult than stomping and yelling.

THERAPIST: Knowing that you have this ability, that you have this new story about yourself, what difference do you think knowing this will make in the next few days and weeks [step 4]?

CLIENT: It will allow me to be more confident that I can do my job and be with my family, without anger messing everything up.

THERAPIST: So it seems to you that you have a way of beating anger that you can rely on in different situations and contexts?

CLIENT: Yes, it might even work with my father.

THERAPIST: Boy, that would really test it, wouldn't it? In the past, anger has been the strongest in that relationship, if I remember correctly.

CLIENT: Yeah, that's for sure! It's been really strong there.

THERAPIST: So you think knowing this about yourself might even enable you to interact with your dad without anger taking over. Do you think you might find yourself doing that in the near future?

CLIENT: Yeah, I'm having lunch with him this week. It would be a good time to start.

THERAPIST: So you plan on using the same strategies that have worked so well . . . like watching for anger's invitations, not trying to convince him of anything, and not taking it personally if he disagrees with you. Is that it?

CLIENT: Yeah, that's the plan. Even if he puts me down, which he almost certainly will.

THERAPIST: You must really be gaining confidence in this new view of yourself, to feel ready for such a step.

CLIENT: Yeah, I guess I am.

Cindy's Case as an Overall Example

The case of Cindy (see text) serves as one of the best examples of all four steps that we have encountered. As the following dialogue demonstrates, no unique outcome is too small to use in the generation of unique redescriptions and possibilities.

THERAPIST: I seem to remember you telling me a story about the first time you realized that you were trying to write a new story for yourself—the one about the soap and the shower. Do you remember?''

CINDY: Yes. I was standing in the shower getting ready to wash myself with the soap in my right hand. I suddenly realized that I didn't have to do it that way, that I could change. So I switched it to my left hand and sort of did it the opposite of how I usually did.

THERAPIST: To many people that might seem a trivial event . . . but for you it wasn't, if I remember correctly.

CINDY: It wasn't trivial at all. It meant I could think about, and change, the habitual way in which I had lived.

THERAPIST: So being able to be aware and switch the soap meant some things?

CINDY: Yes, it meant I could change if I just took the time to think.

THERAPIST: As a result, you slowly but surely began to think about yourself differently—but this was the first breakthrough, the first evidence that it was possible.

CINDY: Yes, that's correct. As small as it was, it still meant that things could be different.

THERAPIST: Gosh, that's an amazing story! How did you manage to pay attention to that small a change, and what do you think it means about you that you did?

CINDY: I'm not sure how I did it. All of a sudden it just happened. As for what it means about me, I think it meant I was ready . . . that no matter how small the steps, I was ready for a new life.

THERAPIST: And the change started by that realization eventually brought you into therapy. Is that correct?

CINDY: Yes, and the changes are still going on.

THERAPIST: What difference do you think knowing all this will make in your future steps?

CINDY: That I can keep taking small steps and get to where I want to go.

Landscapes of Action and of Consciousness

The process described above is based on the narrative notion that stories are not real until they are told, and that the process of getting an account of a story is not a trivial one. The steps we have outlined engage the client in a conversation in which the new story is elicited in a way that renders it both clear and real.

Another way that this process can be conceptualized is in terms of questions that access a client's "landscapes of action" and "landscapes of consciousness" (Bruner, 1990; White, 1991). Landscape-of-action questions can be about the present, past, or future, and invite clients to give accounts concerning actions or behaviors they have engaged in that are at odds with the problem-saturated account. They are particularly useful in obtaining a history of the unique outcome, as well as helping a client to imagine what it might mean in the future. Examples of such questions (White, 1991) are provided below, in addition to those listed above.

• How did you get yourself ready to side with the new story on this occasion? What specific actions did you take to accomplish this?

• Did the old story try to get you not to take such a step? What did you do in order to hold it off?

• How do you think your parents managed to keep their marriage together in the face of trouble's attacks?

Landscape-of-consciousness questions encourage clients to examine the meanings, preferences, commitments, and so forth that might be attached to the unique actions they have identified. These questions invite the clients to render an account concerning "the performance of the alternative preferences, desires, personal and relationship qualities, and intentional states and beliefs, and this culminates in a 're-vision' of personal commitment in life" (White, 1991, p. 31). The following questions serve as examples in this area:

• This new story that you've come to identify with—what does it tell you about what you prefer in your life? About what most appeals to you? About the type of situations and people you are most attracted to?

• Now that you realize that this optional story about you has a history—that it has been around for some time—what does this suggest to you about yourself and what you intend for your life?

• It seems that your son/daughter has struggled for some time to escape the clutches of trouble. What does this suggest to you about what he/she believes to be important in life?

It is suggested that the therapist move back and forth between landscape-of-action and landscape-of-consciousness questions as seems useful. In this way, information about clients' unique behaviors and actions is connected to what these mean about their preferences and desires.

10. Asking Clients the "Miracle Question"

Some Useful Associated Questions

As mentioned in the text, de Shazer, Berg, and their colleagues at the Brief Therapy Center in Milwaukee, Wisconsin have developed a different approach to invite clients to attend to alternate portions of their story (de Shazer, 1988; de Shazer et al., 1986; Berg, 1992; Miller, 1992). Examples of the types of questions they have developed to use in this process are as follows (Miller, 1992):

- When would you say you do not have the complaint? Are there times when it is not present?
- How do you explain the times when the complaint is not present?
- What is different about the times when the complaint is not present?
- What do you imagine that others would say is different when the complaint is not present?
- How is it that things are not worse? What have you managed to do to keep them from worsening?
- What are you doing to keep going when things get really bad?
- How have you been able to survive this situation?
- What will be the first sign that things are getting better?

We have found such questions very useful in obtaining non-problem-saturated accounts from clients. They can be asked as a prelude to the miracle question, or as a means of generating another story without employing the miracle question.

Case Dialogue Example

THERAPIST: So it seems that you are really ready for a change in your life—that this story that has been living you is not getting you what you want. Would this be fair to say?

CLIENT [young adult female]: Absolutely! Things have to change soon. If they don't, I'm not sure what will happen.

THERAPIST: Yes, from your story it's pretty clear that depression has really invaded your life in some major ways. If it continues to control things the way it has, you aren't certain you could continue to stand up to it. You're concerned it might wear you down.

CLIENT: Yes, I'm very concerned about that. I'm getting really tired of it all.

THERAPIST: Almost anyone would be tired of it by now . . . so would it be really important that there be a change?

CLIENT: It would be more important than anything right now.

THERAPIST: So I'm wondering: Suppose there *were* a change? Let's say tonight while you are asleep, something happens, a miracle or something—so that tomorrow when you wake up, the influence of depression will be gone, or at the very least much less. What will be different tomorrow that will let you know that this change has occurred?

CLIENT (*smiling*): Now let me see if I understand—tonight, while I'm asleep, something happens?

THERAPIST: Yes, but since you're asleep, you don't know. But it does, and whatever it is insures that tomorrow depression will be much weaker in your life. What will happen tomorrow that will let you know that this is the case? Let's say the moment that you open your eyes, what will be different?

CLIENT (*still smiling*): Oh . . . I would smile.

THERAPIST: And if you smiled when you first woke up, you would know that depression was weaker?''

CLIENT: Yes.

THERAPIST: What is the next thing that would let you know things are different?

CLIENT: I'd do a little dance across the floor to the bathroom.

THERAPIST: Do you like to sing and dance in the mornings?

CLIENT: Yes, I used to do it all the time.

THERAPIST: But depression doesn't allow that, I bet.

CLIENT: No, it doesn't . . . not at all.

THERAPIST: So you would smile, and then dance and sing. And if you did, that would indicate to you that depression wasn't so much in control—that something had happened to weaken it. Is that right?

CLIENT: Yes, it would be wonderful to start the day like that.

THERAPIST: And what would happen next to let you know things were different? Would there be anything involving other people?

CLIENT: Yes, I would be pleasant with my husband, even if he couldn't be pleasant back. I wouldn't let it affect me so much.

THERAPIST: How would you be more pleasant with him? What would you find yourself doing?

CLIENT: I'd kiss him . . . and (*laughing*) invite him to share my dance with me!

THERAPIST: Gosh, since you have been telling me about this story—the one that would happen if a miracle occurred—you've been laughing and smiling. Do you like this story?

CLIENT: Yes, I like it a lot. It's the way I used to be. I had almost forgotten.

THERAPIST: So this miracle that occurred, you would know it by a return to the way you used to be before depression came along?

CLIENT: Yes, and that would be wonderful!

THERAPIST: Well, I have a suggestion for you, then. Every morning for the next couple of weeks, I suggest that you flip a coin when you open your eyes in the morning. Make this the first thing you do. If it comes up heads, you pretend that the miracle occurred while you slept. If it comes up tails, you pretend that there is nothing different at all.

CLIENT (*with a wrinkled face*): I don't like that!

THERAPIST: What is it you don't like? Help me understand.

CLIENT: I don't want to flip the coin. I want to believe that the miracle has occurred and act accordingly.

THERAPIST: I see. You think that would be more helpful to you?

CLIENT: Yes, definitely.

THERAPIST: Well, you would certainly be a better judge of that than I. So why don't you go ahead and do that? You can let me know how it went in a couple of weeks.

This session proved to be quite powerful in the client's life. It helped her realize that much of depression's influence on her had been tied to her husband's mood and life. Over the subsequent weeks, she made several alterations in this situation, and depression grew weaker accordingly.

It might also be well to note that the "coin flip" intervention is commonly used by de Shazer and Berg in connection with the miracle question. We have found it a very powerful intervention, in that it implies that clients have some control over the stories they live, and that they can alter these if they only "act like" they can. It can also be used without the miracle question, in any context where a client has identified a new story she/he would like to live.

11. Uniting Individuals' Stories with the Stories of Others

The basic intervention for uniting individuals' stories with the stories of other family members is outlined in the body of the chapter. When clients can answer the three questions ("What is my story? What supporting roles do I need? What supporting roles am I willing to play?") then this information is processed in the next session. Often, however, clients will be unable to answer these questions (it is difficult; readers should try it themselves!). In such instances, the therapist explores this difficulty as the basis of the session. The following case dialogue illustrates this process.

THERAPIST (*to husband*): You indicated that you didn't understand the three questions I gave you to look over. How can I help with that?

HUSBAND: Well, I . . . uh . . . I guess I really can't answer what my story is.

THERAPIST: I see. It's not that you don't understand, it's that you find you aren't able to come up with an answer.

HUSBAND: Yes.

THERAPIST: How about the other two questions—about supporting roles you need and roles you are willing to play? Are those equally hard for you to answer?

HUSBAND (*long pause*): Yes, I guess they are.

THERAPIST: So when you ask yourself these questions and look down inside for an answer, you find that you don't have the language for one?

HUSBAND (*looking down at floor*): Yeah, that's about it.

THERAPIST (*to wife*): How about for you? Do you find yourself able or unable to answer the questions?

WIFE: I think I could list things that are important to me, things that I need . . . yes, I think I could answer the first one.

THERAPIST: And the second?

WIFE: Well, I know the supporting role I've been trying to play, but I don't know if it's the one he's been needing. We don't communicate about things like that. I've been guessing all these years.

THERAPIST: So it would have been difficult for you to know what sort of supporting role he needed. If he couldn't tell you, then how would you know?

WIFE: I couldn't . . . and I got tired of playing the one I was after a while.

THERAPIST: How did you know to play the supporting role that you did? If you didn't find out from him, where did you get your information?

WIFE: From my family . . . mainly from my mother. I learned to please others. That's what I tried to do with him for years.

THERAPIST: What happened to your voice in this process?

WIFE: I think it totally got lost. I wasn't aware that it did, but it happened anyway.

THERAPIST: So the way you learned to survive in your family was to be a pleaser, to try and please everyone—everyone but yourself.

WIFE: Exactly, everyone but myself!

THERAPIST: So your role was almost entirely to play supporting roles to others' stories. To do this at the expense of your own story.

IFE: Yes, that's the way it was.

THERAPIST: But a few years ago you received a wake-up call—a call which suggested that this old story had outlived its usefulness for you. At that point you began a process of finding your own story. Is that also accurate?

WIFE: Yes.

THERAPIST: What would you say your husband's child and adolescent survival story was? What did he learn to do in his family?

WIFE: He was the youngest son. All the rest of the children were boys. He didn't have to do anything except be good in school. Around the house, he wasn't required to do anything at all.

THERAPIST (*to husband*): Do you agree with her?

HUSBAND: Yes, for the most part. I was very influenced by my father. My job was to excel in athletics and school.

THERAPIST: Were you asked to play a supporting role to your mom's story? She was the only female in the house. Was she supported?

HUSBAND: No . . . I, uh . . . no, I didn't support her story at all. Not because I didn't want to—it just never entered my mind.

THERAPIST: So the way you survived in your family was to be good at things outside of the home . . . things traditionally male. You were not asked to pay attention or listen to the female voice, it doesn't seem. How would you have learned to do that?

HUSBAND: I wouldn't have . . . I guess I didn't.

THERAPIST: And it seems that part of your childhood story included not sharing your story with women . . . not being asked to. Thus you didn't get much practice at languaging it?

HUSBAND: Yes, I guess so.

THERAPIST: So while you (*to the wife*) were learning how to be a pleaser to survive, you (*to the husband*) were learning how to excel out there in the male world and be taken care of when you came home. I can certainly see how trouble and conflict might have been able to use those stories to gain control of your marriage.

WIFE: Well, they've certainly been able to do that!

12. Family "Talking-Stick" Sessions

The details of family "talking-stick" sessions have been outlined in the text. Included below are examples of questions we have found useful in the processing of the family's experience of these sessions.

- I am interested in how each of you felt during the talking-stick session. Can you describe your experience so that I can understand?
- Did it feel different to be part of the family during these sessions than it does at other times? If so, how? What is your understanding of how this difference came to be?
- What do you think it means about the family that you were able to get together and share pleasant stories and memories? Is there anything that might be important for you to realize about the family because of this?
- Of the stories told in your talking-stick session, which was your favorite? (Let each member respond.)
- Were any of you surprised that your family had shared stories that people could remember? Had trouble and conflict almost gotten you to forget them?
- Can you give me an account of how the family was able to keep trouble and conflict at bay on the occasions represented in your stories? How was it that trouble and conflict didn't manage to take over at these times?
- How is it that your family has been keeping such stories secret lately? Does it make you wonder what other good stories have been going unattended?

13. Family Stories That Control versus Stories That Allow Personal Control

As outlined in the chapter, we have found that all families have stories of both the spoken and unspoken varieties. These can be used both in the process of deconstructing the old story and in story re-vision, as the following example indicates.

THERAPIST: There's one other thing I'd like to suggest: You might find it interesting to remember some of your family stories. Not only remember them, but sort them into those which invited you to conform and those which invited you to be an individual.

CLIENT: You mean the ones I've been living recently.

THERAPIST: No, I meant those of your family of origin—the family you grew up in.

CLIENT: Oh, wow! There were lots of those!

THERAPIST: Yes, I'll bet there were. Would it be interesting to think about which ones would support your conforming to an old story versus which ones would invite you to become an individual?

CLIENT: It was a mixed bag . . . there were both kinds.

THERAPIST: Exactly. Perhaps you could think on it and tell me some of each at our next session?

CLIENT: Yeah, that might be important for me, since I'm living with some of those stories in my house right now! [The client's elderly parents were living with her.]

THERAPIST: Yes, that does make sense. I'll look forward to hearing some of them.

In this particular case, the client had already made considerable progress in the re-vision of her story, but had requested a session in order to be able to better stand up to situations that were inviting her to fall back under the habitual pull of an old story of living her life under the domination of the male voice. This intervention was suggested as a means of rendering the origins of the old story even more visible, as well as providing her with a basis for a further re-vision—a re-vision based upon family stories that would support her further experimentation with the new story she wanted to live.

14. Parenting to Protect versus Parenting to Prepare

We have found the distinction between protective parenting and preparative parenting very useful indeed. It seems that most parents can relate to the differences between these two stances very well. Following are examples of questions we use to explore this area:

• Most parents start out believing that ''Parenting to Protect'' should be the title of their parenting story—and rightly so, as infants are very helpless little creatures. As time progresses, many children ask their parents to switch to a new title, that of ''Parenting to Prepare.'' How much of your parenting these days is informed by parenting to protect as compared to parenting to prepare?

• Which would be most important to you—to parent to protect or to parent to prepare?

• What would be the differences between these two? How would parenting to prepare be different from parenting to protect?

• If we asked your adolescent which he/she needs the most, protection or preparation, what do you think he/she would say? How much protecting would your adolescent need, and how much preparation?

• In your family of origin, did your parents practice parenting to protect or parenting to prepare? Which would you have preferred when you were 16?

• If you wanted to begin parenting to prepare a little more, what steps could you take to try this out and see if you like it?

• In what ways are you already parenting to prepare? Has this proven useful? How have you managed to do this in these areas?

15. Emphasizing Conflicting Stories Rather Than Conflicting People

There are certainly areas in which the distinction between conflicting stories and conflicting people can be used that differ from the parent–adolescent example outlined in the text and in Figure 3.3. It has proven useful when comparing one spouse's story to the story of the other spouse, one family's story to that of another, or one cultural or ethnic group's story to a different group's story. The emphasis of this approach is on the narrative accounts that people have inherited and been influenced by, rather than on the people themselves. Rather than viewing people as acting intentionally or maliciously in relationship to each other, it suggests that people are living out their different stories to the best of their ability, and that the *stories* are colliding, not the *people*. This is in keeping with the narrative theme of this book, which emphasizes the "stories which are living people." Some useful questions for exploring this distinction are as follows:

• If you viewed what is happening in your relationship—the influence that trouble and conflict are managing to have—as depending upon differences in the particular stories you have about the world rather than upon character flaws in each other, would this invite a difference in the way you currently view things? If so, how?

• It seems that both of you came out of your childhood with similar survival stories—that both of you learned to rely on anger to protect yourselves when you feel hurt or threatened. How much of the time in your current marital relationship do you think these old stories control what goes on between you? What sense would you make of the notion that your spouse's cooperation with anger is due more to this childhood survival story than to dislike of you?

• So one of you was raised in a stereotypical Italian home, while the other was being raised in a equally stereotypical Native American environment. To what extent do you feel conflict relies on the differences in these stories to remain strong?

• If you came to see your spouse as trying as hard as she/he can to be true to the story she/he was brought up with, while you are trying to do the same, would that invite you to change the way you interact with your spouse? How?

It should also be emphasized that the telling of these different stories in the therapeutic environment is not a trivial event, in our opinion. Often family members have not unreservedly shared the hopes, fears, and teachings that formed their lives; their understanding of one another can be greatly increased via this process. To come to realize that one's partner acts the way he/she does in the service of protecting himself/herself according to the specifications of a survival story that long predates the present relationship invites one to take things less personally. The hearing of the mate's survival tale can invite some significant changes in the way one reacts to the mate. As emphasized over and over in this work, "Never underestimate the power of a story."

16. Inviting Responsibility via Examining Intentionality

The process of exploring intentionality has been described in the text. Some examples of questions that we use in connection with this process and with the intentionality worksheet (see Figure 3.4) are as follows:

• How are your intentions different in interactions you have experienced as pleasant versus those you have experienced as unpleasant?

• What sorts of intentions usually characterize interactions that you would describe as unpleasant? How old are these intentions—that is, when did you first start getting into such an intentionality? Are such intentions typical of the family you grew up in? Would there be other people who would be similar?

• What have you learned about your spouse's (or child's, friend's, etc.) intentions that you didn't know previously? Which of these surprised you the most?

• Of the intentions that you identified in completing the worksheet, which represent intentions that you would prefer—that are most like the person you want to be?

• What restrains you the most from being in your desired intentionality?

• How much are others in charge of your intentions, and how much are you in charge? What percentage of your intentions are "re-actions," and what percentage are "actions"?

• When you were in an intentionality that might be characterized as protecting yourself (or any other one that the person has selected from the worksheet), what was the outcome that you expected? How did you expect the other person to think, feel, and behave? Did the person behave the way you expected, or differently?

The Therapist and Reflecting Team as Re-Visionary Editors

In the preceding chapter, we have described a form of therapy that utilizes a client's story as a means of providing therapeutic options, with the intent of liberating the person to explore alternative versions of himself/herself. Various examples have been provided of the interviewing process within which the client's story is told and retold in response to various "editorial" questions and reflections by the therapist. This chapter comments further on the role of the therapist as editor. It also discusses the role that a reflecting team can play as an "editorial committee," especially in regard to tracking the hidden text during the session.

We have been stimulated to include such a chapter in response to suggestions and questions raised by our therapist trainees and students over the years. They have sensed that editorial questions and wonderings are an integral part of this type of therapy, and have consistently expressed an interest in having a set of guidelines to help in formulating such questions. They have emphasized (and this matches our experience as well) that being able to generate such questions quickly in the rapid-fire atmosphere of a therapeutic conversation is one of the most challenging aspects of this work. We hope that this chapter will serve to address some of these concerns by documenting the concepts that inform the type of editorial questions we ask when conducting a therapeutic session or serving as a member of a reflecting team.

THE THERAPIST AS RE-VISIONARY EDITOR

To "edit," to paraphrase *Webster's New World Dictionary* (Guralnik, 1982), is to supervise or direct the publication of a newspaper or book; to collect, prepare, and rearrange materials for publication; to revise, omit, or eliminate; or to prepare via deleting, rearranging, and splicing as in a motion picture or television film. An "editor" is one who engages in such processes for a living. As such, editors are very interested in story lines, character development, story composition, the author's motivation or purpose, phrasing and dialogue, and clarity, just to name a few of their concerns. They consistently ask themselves questions such as the following to aid them in their task:

1. Is this the best way the story can be told? What could be changed that would render the story clearer and more understandable for the reader/viewer?

2. Would the story be better served if something were left out? Added? Rearranged?

3. Are the characters believable? Does the reader/viewer have enough information to know what "makes them tick"?

4. Who is the author of the story? What was her/his motivation in writing it the way she/he did? Could another author do a better job?

5. Does this particular story line get across the point of the narrative, or would another version be more useful?

6. How does the plot unfold across time? What characters change, and which ones remain the same?

7. What sort of characters does the narrative contain (happy, sad, violent, etc.)?

8. What are the major obstacles in the story that prohibit the characters from getting what they want? Who is the antagonist? The protagonist?

9. Does any wording or narrative need to be changed so that the story would read better?

In using this metaphor of the therapist as editor, we are suggesting that the therapeutic process can be usefully viewed as being very similar to the description above. That is, the therapy involves the rearranging, cutting and pasting, word processing, and so forth of the client's story, and in this process the therapist/editor works with a story that has already been authored by someone else. From this perspective, the editor's job is not to become the major author, but rather to serve as one who provides space for the client (the major author) to cut, paste, and rearrange the present story such that it suits him/her better. In narrative therapy, this is accomplished by interacting with the client in such a manner that a better story is coevolved in the process of this interaction. We further suggest that the therapist can most usefully provide space for story re-vision through a process in which listening to the client's story is carefully mixed with questioning conducted from an "editorial" stance. In this process the therapist and the client work together, much as an editor and an author might, toward the goal of producing a story that is acceptable to the author. This is an exercise in "visioning and re-visioning" the client's story until it takes on a form that the client agrees is more useful than the one he/she brought to therapy. It involves having narrative conversations about the problem until it is no longer necessary to talk about a problem (Anderson & Goolishian, 1990).

Lest the reader carry this analogy too far, some words of caution seem in order. The therapist/editor is not considered to be quite the expert on story construction and revising that a literary or film editor might be. Instead, the client/author is considered the expert and final authority on her/his story. If the therapist has expertise, it is in the area of wonderings, musings, reflectings, and contrastings that invite the client/author to view his/her story as a narrative that can be changed, rather than as a reality that is fixed in space and time. However, rather than viewing the therapist as an expert on anything, we would suggest that the therapist might better be viewed as an "editorial catalyst." For as Lowe (1991) has succinctly pointed out, to treat postmodern narrative therapy as something sacred, with accompanying disciples, teachers, and masters, is to miss its point completely. The client's voice and the liberation of this voice are what we seek to emphasize in doing therapy from a narrative stance—not the therapist's expertise.

Also, we have become aware that quite often the clients seeking our editorial services have *not* been the major authors of the stories they relate to us in therapy. Much of the time it seems that they have been more "readers" than "writers," and are blindly living out a mythology (a shared story) that they were handed very early in life, as described in previous chapters. Thus a therapist/editor is working not only with a story that he/she has not written, but often with one in which the client has been a marginal author at most. This is also different from a literary or film editor's task. In therapy, it is often necessary to begin the process of the client's becoming her/his own author (as described at length in the preceding chapter). In such instances, the therapist's/editor's job is to be of assistance to this new author until she/he gets the feel for "having pen in hand."

Even in light of these differences, however, the analogy of the therapist as a re-visionary editor has proven to be very useful for us. When we remember that our own stories are not what we are working with, we are more respectful and careful in our treatment of clients and their stories. When we remember that we are hearing interpretations, we are less judgmental.

GUIDELINES FOR THE RE-VISIONARY THERAPIST/EDITOR

In this section we attempt to provide the general guidelines that inform our work as re-visionary editors of clients' stories. These are not new or novel ideas; many readers will no doubt have been exposed to many of them previously. However, we have found them to be ideas that endure, and ones that can be profitably reviewed on a regular basis. Such a review has been beneficial in reminding us of the types of questions we want to ask. We hope that these will, along with the sample questions and dialogues provided in the end-of-chapter appendix, give readers a sufficient basis for experimenting with this model in their own work as therapists.

Editorial Guideline 1: Maintaining Neutrality

The therapist/editor should try to be reasonably neutral, especially in couple or family contexts. This guideline should be violated rarely and only with caution. Readers are referred to Selvini Palazzoli, Boscolo, Cecchin, and Prata (1980) for a complete treatment of this subject. For our purposes, it suffices to say that if therapists are feeling "for someone" or "against someone," or if they have assigned roles or labels to their clients that they believe are "true," they can be reasonably sure that therapeutic neutrality has slipped away. Re-visionary therapists/editors are not much interested in assigning roles or blame to the characters in clients' stories. Rather, they are more interested in how the characters interact, and in how problems may be inadvertently maintained by such interactions. Anderson and Goolishian (1990) have summarized this principle very well in asserting that a therapist needs to be able to "engage in multiple contradictory conversations without invalidating any of them." The therapist/editor considers all stories valid, important, and worthy of being told. This assumption is one of the cornerstones of the narrative interviewing process.

We do not mean to suggest that therapists should be neutral in all situations, or that neutrality implies that all members of a system have contributed equally to a given problem situation. In cases of violence or sexual abuse, our understanding of neutrality does not include holding the victims responsible for their abuse. Instead, we would suggest that once the primary issues of safety have been attended to, therapists need to be interested in the stories of the perpetrators, so that they can perhaps be liberated into a more responsible way of connecting with others. Neutrality is not synonymous with therapist approval; rather, it implies a willingness to listen to stories told from a variety of perspectives.

Editorial Guideline 2: Remaining Curious

The therapist as editor is very curious, but knows very little. A good, albeit humorous, model for this guideline is the television character Columbo as portrayed by Peter Falk (Fisch, Weakland, & Segal, 1982). Put another way, this guideline suggests that the therapist not know much, but always stay willing to find out. A good check for whether therapists are following this guideline is for them to monitor their boredom while conducting therapy sessions. If they find themselves bored, it is a pretty good bet that their curiosity has been put on hold and that they are assuming that they know all that is important about their clients (Stewart, personal communication, 1989). This guideline dovetails very nicely with neutrality, as not knowing invites therapists to remain neutral. Conversely, it is pretty hard to be neutral when therapists are sure that they know something about someone. This guideline has been clarified by Nichols and Schwartz (1991), who have asserted that as therapists we can "know approximations of reality, but we must remain humble about them because of our awareness that they are distorted and incomplete" (p. 147).

Editorial Guideline 3: Being Compassionate

Carl Rogers (1957) is the major source for the third guideline: being compassionate and giving people the benefit of the doubt. Its basis is unconditional positive regard—in this case, trusting that people have the ability to reauthor their stories, and that clients are trying to do just that. This guideline also combines nicely with the previous two. If therapists are neutral and curious, compassion is an easy step away. A good check for whether compassion is present is for therapists to monitor how much resentment, impatience, and frustration they are feeling toward their clients. Compassion and resentment are not common bedfellows.

Editorial Guideline 4: Treating Everything as Information

Everything that happens and is said in therapy can be treated as information in an ongoing story about how therapists can be more helpful in their editorial role (Imber-Black, personal communication, 1985). Rather than labeling certain client behaviors as resistance or denial, therapists can view them as information about how they can posture themselves in order to be more helpful. The same point can be made concerning client symptoms: Instead of focusing upon them literally in order to come up with some "accurate title" for a client's story (such as "The Case of the Paranoid Schizophrenic"), a therapist can ask herself/himself what the client may be trying to communicate that he/she has been unable to get heard in any other way.

For example, when confronted by stereotypically "rigid" parents who find it impossible to treat their 17-year-old daughter any differently from when she was 6, asking what story information is being communicated is very different from making assumptions about the parents, especially negative ones. This sort of thinking leads to curiosity (it should be noted that all of these guidelines mesh together) about the parents have come to feel so strongly about such issues, and to be restrained from entertaining any optional versions of what it means to be parents. It invites the therapist to wonder (*à la* Columbo) about what sort of rules these people have have been taught about what it means to be good parents. Such musings can postpone judgment in the interest of gathering more information.

This can be further illustrated by the story of an adolescent male who came into Doan's therapy room with green, purple, and orange spiked hair; rings in his nose, cheek, and earlobe; and army attire complete with ammo belts and a knife. Doan can still hear Evan Imber-Black's voice whispering into the phone receiver from behind the mirror: "Rob, if you stopped paying so much attention to all the symptoms, and asked yourself what this person is trying to communicate about his life, what sort of questions would you want to ask?"

Editorial Guideline 5: Going with Resistance

Therapists should go with all "resistance" and avoid taking an opponent stance with clients about what sorts of stories they should author (Adler, 1956; Haley, 1973). Often therapists as editors can find themselves invited to join a story and operate according to rules and roles that are already in motion. For example, a therapist can fall prey to trying to convince a set of parents that they should change, in much the same manner that the parents are trying to convince their adolescent offspring to change (and usually with about the same degree of success). Such opponent stances—which invite therapists to convince clients not only that they should re-vision their stories, but also how they should do it—inevitably result in an escalation of the clients' resentment and defensiveness. This often happens when a therapist takes the stance of inadvertently trying to edit a client's story from an "outside expert" stance. The notion of going with resistance implies that therapists should give clients the space and opportunity to author their stories in their own way, even if this includes staying the way they are.

For example, when confronted with a father who presents himself for the first family therapy session with the announcement that he is not going to say a word, a therapist may be tempted to "know" and respond with something like this: "Well, therapy does most of its work through talking, so it is hard for me to understand how anything will be accomplished." Conversely, if the therapist pays attention to this editorial guideline, the response may be as follows: "It's odd you should say that; I've found that people are very unique and different in their responses to situations like this. I'm glad you feel free to know what is best for you."

Editorial Guideline 6: Watching for Strengths

Therapists should constantly be on the alert for their clients' strengths and resources. The manner in which people have already managed to take over the authorship of their lives can provide the therapists with good clues about the types of editorial input that will have the best chance of furthering this reauthoring process. To follow this guideline, a therapist/editor tries to avoid paying more attention to the "problem-saturated" portions of a client's story than to the "solution-saturated" parts (White, 1988b). We have found that it helps to keep in mind that human lives are too diverse and varied to be accurately encapsulated in only one story (Epston, 1989b); such an attempt invariably focuses on certain events at the exclusion of others. The traditional mental health story has focused upon pathology and tragedy at the expense of strengths and resources. From this frame of reference, therapists can sometimes become as overwhelmed as their clients. When this occurs, the sixth guideline can be immensely helpful.

This can be exemplified by a case in which there was a long-distance call from a client during the therapist's summer vacation. This client had been doing very well, but related over the phone that he had gone to a wild party and used a drug that had influenced his life for many years in the past. He was convinced that this proved that he had not improved, and that all his work had been for nothing. When asked whether he was still under the influence of the drug in question, he replied, "Of course not. I would never call you high. I only took one shot." The therapist wondered how it was that the client had found the strength actually to feel the influence of a very powerful old enemy and not to continue using the drug. The client seemed shocked by this twist in the story and began to laugh. It was decided that this was one of his biggest victories over trouble—to face an old monster and then turn and walk away. He agreed that in the past he would not have been able to do this. Focusing on his strengths rather than his weaknesses seemed quite useful to him in continuing his new story.

Editorial Guideline 7: Expanding the Focus

When the story is not making sense, the focus should be expanded (Imber-Black, personal communication, 1985). This guideline takes an opposite view from the traditional Western/mechanistic manner of thinking, which suggests that when one is confused, the best course is to be reductionistic. There is a strong, historically dominant story in our culture that true understanding involves being able to reduce something to its most essential elements. This can be a very useful model for many areas of interest, but in dealing with the problems that humans encounter in the process of living, a wide-angle lens is often more useful. Stories about problems, symptoms, meanings, and ideas sometimes only make sense when viewed from a larger editorial context that includes how the problem-saturated story has evolved in relation to larger systems (religious background, family tradition, ethnic heritage, etc.). When a reductionistic approach is taken, therapists can often miss the dominant meanings and knowledges that inform the thinking of the people in question. When the larger cultural stories and themes that have been a significant part of the clients' lives are included, new understandings and further curiosity will usually result.

A case that illustrates the usefulness of this guideline was that of a young husband who seemed to have lost all sexual and emotional interest in his wife. This loss coincided with the couple's discovering that the wife was unable to have children. The therapist and the team involved in the case were strongly invited to view this young man as selfish, insensitive, and patriarchal. There was some confusion about this, however, as he maintained that he loved his wife and did not wish to divorce her. In expanding the focus, it was discovered that he was under a great deal of pressure from his parents to have a son. This expanded version of the narrative, and what it revealed about the dilemma the young man was in, was very useful to the therapist in following all the editorial guidelines we have mentioned, as well as providing better information about how to proceed in the case.

Editorial Guideline 8:
Giving Oneself Permission "Not to Know"

Re-visionary therapists/editors should give themselves permission "not to know," as well as to take breaks during sessions, consult with colleagues about cases, and read what others have done in similar circumstances. It is very rare that good stories get written entirely in the first draft. It is far more common for there to be "writes and rewrites," in which therapists and clients learn as much about what the clients do not want to say as what they do. Our trainees tell us that one of the most helpful suggestions we offer is to be sure to make at least three mistakes in each session! Not only do editors seldom encounter the perfect story; the editing job usually takes some revising as well.

A useful exercise in this regard is for therapists to take a break from sessions that they are experiencing as difficult, and ask themselves how other therapists that they know well would view the case. What would they see differently? What other types of information would they be interested in gathering? Often this will create openings that can be explored. It can also be useful for therapists to tell clients that they need a couple of days to think about the clients' stories—and then actually take the time to do so. Such a break can be followed up by sending a therapeutic letter that contains new observations and questions for a client or family to consider (letter writing is covered in a subsequent chapter).

Editorial Guideline 9:
Not Working Harder Than Clients

Therapists should try not to work harder at re-visioning the clients' stories than the clients are working themselves. Usually no change will occur while this is happening (Bergman, 1985; Berg, 1992), although much of the traditional training that those of us in the helping professions receive would have us believe that this should be a major part of our job description!

Therapists and clients can often get caught in a loop similar to those that occur between parents and children. The harder the therapists work, the less hard the clients are invited to work; the more responsible the therapists become, the less responsible the clients are invited to become; and so on and so forth. The caring but overly responsible therapist is an easy mark for this type of interaction. "Working Harder Than My Clients" is also an excellent title for a story whose final chapter will be "Burned Out."

Editorial Guideline 10:
Focusing on What Symptoms Depend Upon

Instead of focusing on the symptoms that are prominent in a client's narrative, a therapist should focus on what the symptoms depend upon in order to stay in existence. This guideline is based upon cybernetic thinking, and assumes that the behaviors storied as symptoms do not occur in isolation, but rather are maintained by some standard or set of meanings that issues invitations for the symptomatic behaviors to continue. The symptoms that are commonly understood as depression provide an excellent example. In order for a person to be participating in a story where she/he is playing a character who feels helpless, hopeless, and self-depreciative, it is usually necessary that there be some standard or set of meanings that "calls forth" these sorts of thoughts and feelings. Perfectionism, or some other unattainable standard, is a likely candidate in such circumstances. When a person is caught up in a long-standing story in which perfectionism defines the way she/he must be, then failure and the feelings and thoughts that usually accompany it are almost inevitable outcomes. Depression thrives on such a story, and can "grow fat" when unrealistic goals are present.

Editorial Guideline 11:
Asking "What Would It Mean" Questions

Therapists should remember to ask "what would it mean" questions regularly when conducting interviews. This is another way of saying that it is often useful to ask clients what sort of assumptions or premises form the basis of their current stories. In our experience, most people (therapists included) are largely unaware of the assumptions that inform their thinking. These usually remain unexamined, and as such are a potential portion of the hidden text. Questions that explore such meaning systems can provide re-visionary therapists/editors with useful information about how their clients think, reason, and behave.

For example, upon encountering a mother who seems to be unable to change her habit of protecting her son from the consequences of his behavior, asking "What would it mean if you let your son experience the consequences of failing and having to repeat a class at school?" may provide useful information. Her response may reveal that such an action on her part would mean that she is no longer a caring parent, or that she has failed as a parent. Other possible responses may include her being accused by her parents of not caring, or blamed by her husband for letting their son down. Such information supplies the therapist with a view into the rules and meanings that inform this client's behavior.

We have also found meaning questions to be very helpful when clients come in with diagnostic labels they have been given by other therapists and helpers. Instead of simply assuming that such labels are not helpful, we have found it more useful to ask these clients for their understanding of what their particular labels mean. If they indicate that the labels have been useful and enabling, then we are invited to "work with" them rather than change them. If, however, they indicate that the labels have been very impoverishing and have invited them to feel powerless, we then seek alternate meanings that are more empowering.

This can be illustrated by the cases of two clients, both of whom had been diagnosed as manic–depressive or bipolar. In response to questions about what this label meant to them, two very different stories emerged. In one instance the client felt helpless, hopeless, and beaten down by being so labeled. It was understood that bipolar illness was an incurable disease about which nothing could be done except take medications, which created unpleasant side effects. In response to this meaning construction, we began to talk about the influence of an "up-and-down lifestyle" and to draw distinctions about the areas in the client's life that it had been unable to steal away. In the second case, the client felt quite differently about the label. It replaced words like "schizophrenic" and "crazy," and opened the door for a medication that could be used as part of a solution. Our response to this meaning construction was to keep the label and to talk about medication as one strategy that was proving helpful. This illustrates our belief that the client's meanings rather than the therapist's are important. Thus, many of our questions are informed by this line of thinking.

Editorial Guideline 12:
Maintaining a Gender-Sensitive Stance

Therapists need to make every effort to maintain a gender-sensitive stance that recognizes the validity of both the female and the male voices. This guideline suggests that we keep in mind that each of us looks through a "gender lens" (Hoffman, 1990), which invites us to view the world from a particular point of view. Care is required if a therapist is to escape the biases and prejudices that accompany stereotypical gender stories.

Gender is one of the most powerful and dominant stories informing our personhood. Each of us has been highly influenced by the specifications and notions associated with being of a particular gender. It is our experience that a gender-sensitive stance is an absolute necessity in the arena of family therapy; without it, the therapist will be at a distinct disadvantage. Again, in using the term "gender-sensitive," we mean to imply a stance that views both genders as equally valid or mutual, rather than one that invites a "one-up" stance (so common in this area).

THE REFLECTING TEAM
AS AN EDITORIAL COMMITTEE

General Guidelines

The notion of using a "reflecting team" in therapy was introduced by Tom Andersen (1987), and since that time has become quite a popular idea among certain groups of family therapists. Such a procedure involves having a team observe a therapy session (usually from behind a one-way window) and then allowing the team the opportunity to discuss and wonder about the therapeutic conversation, with the therapist and family becoming the observers to this discussion. The theoretical basis of Andersen's ideas can be found in the work of Gregory Bateson (1972, 1978, 1980) and Humberto Maturana (1978), both of whom have suggested that reality is created by the observer, and that problems are encountered when different observers come into conflict over which version of reality is the "true and correct" one. However, when different versions of reality are simply shared, rather than being presented as true and correct, room for perceptual change is often created. The reflecting team's purpose is to provide a sharing of differing perspectives, in the hope that this will invite the therapist and the family to entertain alternate versions of reality that will prove less problematic to the family members than those they held previously. In order to insure that the team's ideas are understood as differing perspectives, rather than as recommendations for the way the family should be, the following guidelines have been suggested by Lynn Hoffman (1989):

1. Descriptions and observations are best delivered from a stance of mutual positive regard.

2. Symmetrical escalations are to be avoided. "Both–and" statements are preferable to "either–or" statements. The introduction of new ideas should be preceded by a comment of appreciation.

3. Reflections are not supervision or problem solving; rather, they should be phrased tentatively, in hypothetical language ("perhaps," "maybe," "if," etc.)

4. Team members should be careful about siding with one member of the family via leaving other people out, or pointing the finger at certain members of the family. If one member is praised it is best to praise them all.

5. It is better to make observations at the systemic level, via the use of stories, metaphors, and analogies that access meanings rather than behaviors. Whatever is said should be empowering rather than demeaning.

6. Reflections should be made to other members of the team rather than to the family or therapist. The family and therapist should "overhear" them. This allows the family members more freedom to accept or reject what they are hearing, and invites them to feel less as if someone is trying to "fix" them.

7. In teams of three or four persons, it is usually best to limit reflections to two major ideas per person, with the total time for reflections limited to between 5 and 10 minutes.

8. It is best if the team does not share thoughts behind the mirror, as it is important that each voice be a "personal" one.

9. What is said is most useful if it is a description rather than a prescription. Emphasis on "an idea of what is" is preferable to "what is."

10. There are no correct statements or errors. The family members decide which of the reflections are most useful for them.

11. Position rather than hierarchy is emphasized, and the integrity of everyone's position is respected.

12. Reflections can be similar to those of a Milan-style team (making hypotheses, looking for themes, suggesting rituals, etc.), but these are given in the form of tentative questions and wonderings rather than assignments.

Zimmerman (1992) has stressed that the use of reflecting teams has accompanied a desire on the part of therapists to become more "transparent" in their work with clients. To further this process, he has suggested that team members also invite one another to "situate" their comments and wonderings during the reflecting session. In other words, the team members can ask one another to explain their responses by situating them in theoretical ideas, imagination, or their own experience. This allows the clients to know where the various team members "are coming from," and is thus more transparent. He further suggests that upon occasion, the reflecting team can be invited into the session for the purpose of asking the therapist questions along with the clients. This invites the therapist to be totally open, and to be able to say things that otherwise might go unsaid. It allows the therapist to situate his/her comments and observations as well.

We concur with these general guidelines for a reflecting team's work, and have been very interested in including the use of such a team in our own clinical practice. In the remainder of this section, we present some thoughts on the use of a reflecting team that can be used in addition to those already given.

Using the Reflecting Team
to Track the Hidden Text

In our work, we have come to view the reflecting team as an "editorial committee," which further extends the notion of the therapist as editor. In serving this function, the team members strive to remain aware of the therapist-as-editor suggestions previously presented, as well as the general guidelines for the reflecting team's participation. To these notions we add the additional idea of asking the team members to be responsible for tracking the "hidden text" (see Chapter 2), so that the therapist can remain free simply to elicit, and listen to, the client's story. That is, we ask our team members to be attentive to that which is not said (the "unspeakable"), which is often connected to a client's greatest fear.

In our experience, this unspoken hidden text is often connected to the primal fear of rejection and abandonment (which is connected to the feeling that one is not good enough to be lovable—i.e., shame). This fear has a high potential to develop during the vulnerable childhood and adolescent years. Issues as deep and as threatening as rejection and abandonment are often dealt with in childhood via either a "fight" or "flight" response. This choice can form one of the major elements of the childhood survival story, and develops as the habitual manner in which the person attempts to protect herself/himself from the threat of rejection, disapproval, and (at the extreme) abandonment. The "fight" response manifests itself as the tendency to react to threatening situations via acting out, confrontation, and anger. The "flight" response is demonstrated by those who habitually rely on avoidance and retreat. Both of these survival stories have in common the capacity to allow a person to survive childhood without coming to terms with the fear of rejection and disapproval. As a result, this fear can remain unspoken and become a major portion of the hidden text. The outcome is that many of a person's behaviors, whether they are characterized by anger or avoidance, become the unspoken part of the plot of a prevailing story that seeks to avoid confronting or dealing with the greatest fear (rejection/disapproval). As previously pointed out, however, this actually serves to insure that the greatest fear will probably come to pass.

The workings of this process can be illustrated by the lives of people who consistently react to potentially hurtful situations (or situations that they erroneously tell themselves will be hurtful) with anger. Such people (quite often males) come from a childhood story in which anger was employed to survive. This survival technique not only allowed them to keep people at a distance and somewhat off guard, but also enabled them to avoid admitting and dealing with the hurt and pain they were feeling. Caught up in such a story, they habitually showed hurt as anger—a "righteous anger" that allowed them to escape feeling vulnerable as the result of rejection or disapproval. In such a story, hurt remains unspoken; the fear of rejection remains unaddressed; and anger becomes a protective lifestyle. Such an account can actually serve a type of survival value when persons are young and without the option of leaving the "field of play." However, this story commonly outlives its usefulness and begins to become problematic in the persons' lives and relationships as they enter late adolescence and young adulthood.

When a client who is being lived by such a childhood survival story presents for therapy, the narrative that the therapist and reflecting team usually hear is one of rebellion, resentment, hostility, self-damaging acting out, and extreme anger. The underlying hurts, fears, and vulnerabilities that fuel such feelings remain largely unspoken. The client may even be unaware that such feelings exist, or at the very least is reluctant to discuss them. Rather, the anger so often expressed can be seen as the primary actor in a story designed to avoid such an admission, as well as the pain and vulnerability that are likely to accompany it. Paradoxically, the regular expression of anger insures that such a client's greatest fear, that of rejection and disapproval, will consistently come to pass as others find themselves unwilling to be in anger's presence. In the model of therapy that we are suggesting, the reflecting team's function is to offer editorial wonderings about this unspoken portion of the story—musings that invite the client to explore addressing the hurt in his/her life in more useful ways than cooperating with anger.

In the survival story characterized by withdrawal, anxiety, or shyness, a different type of protection is used. The story that develops is one of habitual avoidance of situations in which displeasure, disapproval, or rejection might be encountered, rather than one of acting out in righteous indignation. In most such stories, each episode of withdrawal accomplishes the short-term outcome of anxiety reduction, which serves to reinforce the avoidant response further. This reduction in anxiety is connected not only to the avoidance of the threatening relationship situation, but to the avoidance of facing the greatest fear of rejection/abandonment. Like the survival story characterized by anger, such a story can often serve a useful protective function during the childhood and adolescent years (via inviting others to play a superprotective role, to name only one). However, this type of story also tends to begin to outlive its usefulness in late adolescence and adulthood, as the avoidant behavior renders it less and less likely that the persons can successfully complete the developmental steps of these periods. The consistent avoidance serves to insure that the persons will not gain the approval they so desperately desire; instead, they will be controlled by a story in which they are unable to get what they want and are consistently rejected. Not only that, but avoidance stories are typically developed at the expense of the persons' learning how to exercise their own voices or become their own authors. The consistent avoidance insures that they will sacrifice their voices and experiences in the service of not risking rejection. This can lead to a growing sense of self-erasure as these persons move into the adult developmental period.

Therapists and reflecting teams exposed to such stories invariably hear an account in which fear of the opinions of others is the dominant issue. Fear and the chance of disapproval dominate such narratives, rather than being unspoken, as in the anger story. Instead, what remains unspeakable is the notion that the clients are not strong enough to survive even the slightest hint of rejection; that they still feel like vulnerable 5-year-olds; and that they have no stories about themselves as competent adults. The unspeakable in such stories is often that they are unlovable and unworthy of others' affections or approval. In such instances, the members of the reflecting team offer wonderings about such unspoken content as consistently as they offer wonderings about the spoken content of the session. Such reflections invite clients to begin deconstructing their old stories which have them playing a role that can be described as a ''vulnerable-little-girl/little-boy lifestyle.''

Since the therapist is relying on the reflecting team to track the hidden text, we have found it useful for the therapist to ask questions that will be helpful in providing this type of information for the team. These are questions that invite clients to consider and comment on aspects of their stories that are commonly not spoken. The prime example of such a question, and one that we have found very useful, is ''What is your greatest fear?'' Examples of other questions of this type, as well as examples of team reflections, can be found in the end-of-chapter appendix.

Other Ideas for Using Reflecting Teams

We have recently started experimenting with being more flexible and creative in our use of the reflecting team from a narrative stance. Although this experimentation is still in its early stages, we describe it here in hopes that readers will find it interesting and will use it to generate new ideas of their own. In addition to using reflecting teams in the manner previously outlined, we have done the following:

1. We have used the team as a literal source of multiple stories. That is, team members are encouraged to construct stories about clients, and then to exchange these stories with one another during the reflecting segment of the session. After this has occurred, the therapist and clients briefly discuss the clients' responses to the various stories. Using a team in this manner models the process of story

re-vision and demonstrates that many different perspectives can be constructed from the same sequence of events. Examples of the types of questions that the therapist can ask in this process are provided in the appendix.

2. We have sometimes sent clients home with reflections that have been written by the team, rather than sharing these reflections with them during the session. We have been becoming increasingly concerned that the reflecting experience can sometimes be very overwhelming to clients, and that many reflections may ''get lost.'' This procedure renders it unnecessary for the clients to remember the reflections, and provides them with the opportunity to ponder them at their leisure. Their thoughts and responses can then be processed in the next session.

3. We have had the team members tell open-ended stories, and invited clients to supply the endings (or the next chapters) for themselves. This procedure invites clients to engage in a ''teleography'' (Howard, 1992)—that is, a telling of their stories based upon future possibilities, rather than constructed it in the standard autobiographical fashion.

4. We have invited the team members into the therapy room for open discussions with the therapist. This includes the team's asking the therapist to be very ''transparent'' in clients' presence—that is, asking the therapist to share why he/she asked particular questions, or what domains of knowledge or theories were informing his/her thinking. The team members invite clients to ask questions of the therapist as well (Zimmerman, 1992). Using a reflecting team in this manner is in keeping with the current trend of ''collaborative'' therapy—a therapy that is open and honest, and that models in every possible manner the notion that therapists and clients can coconstruct what happens between them.

APPENDIX: THERAPEUTIC EXAMPLES

Guidelines for the Re-Visionary Therapist/Editor

Editorial Guideline 1: Maintaining Neutrality

We have found that being intensely interested in hearing each client's story is very useful in allowing a therapist to maintain a neutral stance. Our experience has been that when each person's story has been revealed, the therapist can usually come to an understanding concerning the forces and situations that influenced them along the way. Conversely, when only "one side" of a situation has been heard, the therapist is invited to move away from neutrality. For example, when listening to a wife's story that she is tired of "raising four children" (when there are only three actual children in the house, with the fourth one being her husband), it is very easy to be "for" the wife and to story the husband as patriarchal and irresponsible. When the husband's story is told, however, the therapist may discover that he comes from a background in which "little-boy behavior" has been both expected and supported, and that there have been very few instances of people believing that he is capable of responsible behavior. Instead of being for or against anyone in such an instance a therapist taking, a neutral stance can see both parties as being lived by stories that they learned early in their lives. Harold Goolishian (Anderson & Goolishian, 1990) stated this principle very succinctly when he responded to a question about what he would do if confronted with a client who he thought was a "son of a bitch." He indicated that he would engage such a client in a conversation (hear the story), at the end of which he would no longer feel the need to think about the client in such terms. We agree that one of the cornerstones of neutrality is the willingness to hear all clients' stories from a stance that is consistently open to an altered view of them.

Some Useful Questions for Therapists to Ask Clients

We have found questions that include both sides of a cybernetic pattern to be very useful in maintaining therapeutic neutrality, as well as inviting clients to consider their individual part in any relationship. Examples of such questions are as follows:

• Which would be harder—for your husband to grow up and assume more responsibility in the family, or for you to believe that he can and invite him to do so? Which of you would have a harder time believing that he could become more responsible?

• Which of you is more convinced that your version of things is the correct one? Which of you would be more willing to alter your perception so that a compromise would be more likely?

• If I made an attempt to understand everyone's story in the family equally, would that be OK with everyone? Who would be most upset if I treated everyone's story with equal validity?

Tips for Maintaining Neutrality

• Everyone in the session should be given equal "air time"—that is, a reasonably equal opportunity to tell his/her story.

• A therapist who compliments one person should compliment them all.

• A therapist should not enter into keeping secrets with one member of a family. (Our suggestion in this regard is to have a rule that the therapist is free to share or not to share information, as seems clinically useful to her/him.)

• The therapist should be genuinely interested in each person's story as containing useful information.

Some Useful Questions for Therapists to Ask Themselves

Neutrality is not an easy stance to maintain. Therapists all have their own stories that inform their view of the world. We have found that for a therapist to remain even reasonably neutral, he/she must consistently entertain questions that invite a neutral view. Examples of some of these are as follows:

• Do I believe that the sharing of stories within an accepting atmosphere is probably healing in and of itself? If so, shouldn't I be sure to get everyone's stories told—the "whole" stories?

• Do I have a negative label or story about this client? What sort of information do I need to gather to invite an alternate version of her/him?

• If, instead of viewing this client as stubborn or resistant, I saw the client as being scared, how would my story about him/her change?

• If, instead of viewing the members of this family as "wanting to be unhappy," I understood them to be "restrained from being different," what difference would that make in my thinking about them?

• If I were more sensitive to the situation of my clients, and less married to a model of therapy, what might change in my story about them?

• If I spent as much energy in listening to everyone's viewpoint as I have in disliking the wife/husband in this family, what might I learn that has previously gone unseen?

• What sort of story does the diagnostic label that has been applied in this case by others invite the family members and the therapist to participate in?

Editorial Guideline 2: Remaining Curious

We cannot overemphasize the importance of remaining curious while conducting therapy from a narrative stance. When curiosity disappears, it is most usually replaced with "knowledge"—in other words, stories therapists have constructed about their clients, which they consistently pretend are true and accurate. We recommend that therapists operate from a stance that is characterized by a "question mark" rather than a "period," especially in relation to their clients. We have found this a very liberating guideline, in that it suggests that our job as therapists is "not to know." Accordingly, we ask questions that invite both ourselves and our clients to an exploration of alternate understandings. Consider this example:

CLIENT: I don't want to talk about my sex life. That's not why I'm here. I won't answer any questions about that.

[At this point, the therapist could have told himself a story in which the client was being "resistant," and could have concluded that the sexual area of the client's life must be just filled with "hang-ups," However, the therapist took a curious stance, suspending any "knowing" in the interest of finding out.]

THERAPIST: I appreciate you letting me know that. I will certainly respect your wishes in that area and not ask you anything specific concerning your sex life. Before we move on to areas which you feel would be more useful, can you help me understand how it is that you feel so strongly about this one?

CLIENT: The last therapist I had only wanted to talk about sex. I don't see that as the problem, but I got labeled as the problem anyway. I got accused of not wanting sex often enough. But the relationship I have with my spouse didn't get talked about in any other way. To me, that is the problem . . . if the relationship was good, the sex thing would take care of itself.

THERAPIST: So in your last therapy you felt blamed for the problem, and sex was used as the way to blame you?

CLIENT: That's the way it felt to me.

THERAPIST: And your view of the problem is that it's much more relational than sexual?

CLIENT: Yes . . . it's more about trust.

THERAPIST: So it would be more useful to you if we talked about what restrains you from trusting your spouse than what restrains you from having sex?

CLIENT: Yes. If trust were there, the sex wouldn't be an issue.

Such a conversation certainly invited the therapist into a different story from the "resistant" one. In our experience, our clients usually have very good reasons for thinking and feeling the way they do. Curiosity allows the therapist to explore these stories, rather than siding with a premature and inaccurate one.

Editorial Guideline 3: Being Compassionate

Most therapists would probably agree that having compassion for the client is an essential part of the therapeutic relationship. However, in some instances this is far easier said than done. The therapist's gender, ethnic group, religious orientation, and past experiences can stand in the way of successfully assuming a compassionate stance.

Doan regularly teaches classes in family counseling in which he assigns the movies *The Great Santini* and *The Prince of Tides* for his students to watch and evaluate. One of the most problematic areas for the students is developing compassion for every family member represented in the films. For example, those readers familiar with *The Great Santini* will have no problem understanding why many of the students—especially the female students—find it difficult to feel compassionately about Bull Meecham, the macho, hard-driving, Marine fighter pilot who runs his family like a military unit. When discussing *The Prince of Tides*, the same problem occurs with Lilah, a mother who is determined to raise her social station in life no matter what the cost to certain family members.

Developing the ability to remain compassionate, regardless of one's personal feelings, can be quite a difficult task indeed. Therapists can ask themselves:

* Do I understand that I do not have to "approve" of this person's actions in order to compassionately listen to her/his story?
* If I understood the outside influences that have impacted this client's life, would I be inclined to feel more compassion for him/her?
* What are the possible positive motivations or intentions this client might have? Is she/he a caring person according to her/his definition of "caring"? Is she/he caring in a manner that is hard for me to understand?
* Can I engage this client in a conversation and be willing to change my view of him/her as a result, or is my mind made up? If the latter, what issues in my own life contribute to my "certainty" about this client?

Editorial Guideline 4:
Treating Everything as Information

Case Dialogue Example

In the case of the adolescent male with army fatigues, ammo belts, and so on (see text), the following conversation resulted from being invited to view his appearance as "information":

THERAPIST: You seem to be dressed in a manner which suggests that you need to protect yourself. Is this accurate or am I off base?

CLIENT: No, that's accurate. If you don't defend yourself, people will take advantage of you.

THERAPIST: So dressing and looking this way enables you to feel safer?

CLIENT: Well, some.

THERAPIST: But not completely . . . the fear is still pretty strong?

CLIENT: Yeah.

THERAPIST: And where is this fear the strongest? Where do you feel the most vulnerable?

CLIENT: At home, when I'm in my room. I have lots of things to defend me there.

THERAPIST: So fear is strong when you're alone in your room. What does it look like?

CLIENT: It's big and dark. It can be very powerful.

THERAPIST: And does it have a gender? Is it male or female?

CLIENT: Yeah . . . it's male and it's big.

This line of questioning led to the discovery that the client had been physically abused by his father, and that the hairstyle and clothes he had started wearing invited the father to have less to do with him. Entertaining the notion that his appearance was communication resulted in a very different line of inquiry from that which would have issued from the notion that his appearance was a problem.

Some Useful Questions for Therapists to Ask Themselves

• What are the family members trying to say that they find impossible to say in less symptomatic ways?
• What feeling does this client's behavior/appearance suggest—fear, hurt, anger, sadness, self-depreciation, or something else?
• If I viewed almost everything that clients say and do as trying to communicate something, would I be more interested in understanding or judging?
• Does this client's behavior/appearance suggest a possible childhood survival story that is still strong? If the client were highly influenced by a story out of childhood or adolescence, would this behavior/appearance make sense?

Editorial Guideline 5: Going with Resistance

The fifth guideline reminds us not to be "violent" with our clients. By "violent" we refer to Maturana's (1978) notion of violence, which can be paraphrased as holding an opinion to be true and demanding that another hold it so too. Amundson and Steward (1993) have framed this as the "colonization" of clients' experiential territory, and has suggested that the antidotes to such colonial tendencies are curiosity and uncertainty. We would agree, and add that going with apparent "resistance" rather than confronting it is useful as well. It avoids running the risk of cooperating with an oppositional cybernetic in which the therapist tries harder and harder to convince the client of something while the client works harder and harder at avoiding this acceptance. We have consistently found that oppositional stances do not enhance or facilitate the therapeutic process.

Case Dialogue Example

The following extreme example is offered:

CLIENT: I don't want to be here. The only reason that I'm here is because of the court. I think it's a waste of time, but it beats staying in jail.

THERAPIST: It's funny you should say that. When I got assigned this case, I found myself feeling much the same way. I felt as if I was being forced to talk to someone who probably didn't want to talk to me . . . so I can at least partially understand how you would feel it a waste of time. I'd like to thank you for being so honest with me. Since we both sort of feel forced to be here, can you think of anything useful we could do with the time?

CLIENT: No, not really.

THERAPIST: Perhaps if we just forgot about the notion of doing therapy . . . would you rather drive down to McDonald's and have a Coke?

CLIENT: It would beat just sitting around here.

THERAPIST: I agree *(Heading for the door)* What are your favorite hobbies?

Rather than trying to talk the client into "doing therapy," it proved more useful to allow the client to be resistant, and to focus on establishing a relationship. Drinking Cokes and talking about hobbies led to discussions about the client's life, hopes, and dreams. Therapy can be done at McDonald's!

Some Useful Questions for Therapists to Ask Themselves

• Am I feeling oppositional with this client? Am I invited into a game of "winning and losing" with him/her?

• What sense do I make of the statement that ''there are no resistant clients; there are only restrained ones''?

• If I saw this client's reluctance in therapy as evidence that the therapeutic relationship is not sufficiently strong enough for her/him to feel safe, what would I want to do?

• Is it possible that the members of this family know more about the rate of change that would be good for them than I do? If they did, would I want to know that?

Editorial Guideline 6: Watching for Strengths

Case Dialogue Example

THERAPIST: What happened, John?

CLIENT: Man, I blew it! Anger took me over again. He pissed me off and I hit him!

THERAPIST: So anger managed to sneak up on you and take over?

CLIENT: Yeah . . . man, it's all been for nothing! I thought I was getting better but I'm not. I can't change, everything has been a fake.

THERAPIST: Yeah, I can see how it would feel like that to you, but I'm curious about some things. How is it you aren't still out of control? In the past you'd still have been yelling and screaming, probably cursing me out too. How were you able to get control back from anger so quick this time?

CLIENT: Man . . . I don't know . . . after I hit him I just stopped. I realized what I had done. I just sort of froze up and stopped.

THERAPIST: In a few minutes, the teachers are going to find out about this and ask you to go to time-out a while. Are you going to argue with them like you would have in the past, or are you going to remain in control of anger and go quietly?

CLIENT: No, I'll go quietly . . . in fact, let's just go on down there and I'll put myself in.

THERAPIST: Wow, really? You certainly seem to have given anger the slip a lot faster this time. I understand it got the better of you and got you to hit someone . . . but it sounds like you are going to try and cut your losses to it.

CLIENT: Yeah, no sense making it any worse.

THERAPIST (*as they head for the time-out room*): What do you think it means about you that you are willing to handle this situation so differently from the past?

Some Useful Questions for Therapists to Ask Themselves

• Am I just as prone to overlook small changes in my clients as family members are in each other? Do I want to be?

• Who is being influenced more in therapy? Am I influencing the clients, or are they influencing me? Am I falling prey to the same story (and accompanying symptoms) that they are? Are they convincing me to feel hopeless and overwhelmed?

• My job is to be able to get into a client's frame of reference; do I want it to control me once I have done this?

• Which am I more interested in—pathology or resources? Where do I want to focus more of my energy and attention?

• Have I been able to avoid being invited to be totally responsible for my clients during the last week? Do I believe they are capable, competent people, or do I see them as being dependent and unable to function without me? If I view them as dependent, is this because I am overlooking their strengths and resources?

• How many people in my clients' histories have treated them as if they could be competent, successful people? Do I want to be one of the first to do so?

Editorial Guideline 7: Expanding the Focus

The seventh guideline invites us to look at the dominant themes and stories that inform people's lives. Examples of these are gender, race, religion, family tradition, religious orientation, and nationality, to name a few. When cases are inviting us to be confused, we have found that exploring such areas can often yield information from which a clearer understanding is possible. Put simply, this is a search for the outside factors and forces that often influence and define the problems people are experiencing.

Some Useful Questions for Therapists to Ask Clients

• If you had allowed Eddie to call you a son of a bitch and not hit him, would anyone in your family have been upset with you? Would anyone have told you that you can't let people get away with that sort of thing?

• If you were able to love without worrying about others all the time, would you be breaking any rules about what it means to be a good woman?

• You say that depression's onset was just after you got divorced. How many other people in your family/religion have been divorced? Are you one of the few? The first one?

Case Dialogue Example

HUSBAND: We are afraid our son may be an alcoholic. We don't believe however, that alcholics are born that way. We are here to find out how to change him.

THERAPIST: Let me be sure I understand. How is it that you don't believe alcoholism can be caused by genetics? Can you share that with me so I can understand? Where does that belief come from?

MOTHER: God wouldn't make somebody sin, so he wouldn't create an alcoholic. That wouldn't be fair.

THERAPIST: And would everyone in your family and extended family hold the same belief?

FATHER: Oh yes, absolutely.

THERAPIST: So if you believed that alcoholism can be caused genetically, you would not only be breaking your religious convictions, but you would be departing from a very strong family tradition as well?

MOTHER: Yes, I suppose so, but it's not really the family's belief, it's the word of God.

THERAPIST: Thank you for your very open and candid answers. That really helps me understand how it is you would be so upset about the possibility of your son being an alcoholic. I appreciate that.

MOTHER: You're welcome.

In this example, the issue is not whether the therapist agreed or disagreed with the parents' view of things; the issue is that the therapist understood the larger context in which their view had been formed, and the interpersonal implications of changing this view. With this information in hand, the therapist was invited to view the parents' beliefs in a much more compassionate and understanding manner.

Some Useful Questions for Therapists to Ask Themselves

• Do I have a good understanding for the dominant themes and stories that inform this client's/family's life? Things like religion, race, tradition, gender, and so on?
• Have I invited the members of this family to tell me any family stories? If I asked them to share the stories that they feel would tell me the most about them, what might I learn?
• Do I have a genogram of this family that accounts for at least the last

three generations? Would I be willing to do a session in which such information is gathered?

Editorial Guideline 8:
Giving Oneself Permission "Not to Know"

The eighth guideline has been one of the most liberating ones for us personally. Most of us are trained that "to know" and to be expert are both necessary to do our job well. We would like to suggest exactly the opposite— that *not* knowing is actually more useful in aiding the therapist to maintain a respectful editorial stance in relationship to the client's story. This guideline dovetails very well with that of being curious; not knowing invites curiosity in the quest for more information. Therapists can ask themselves:

- Am I falling prey to the old story that it is my job to supply this client with all the answers? Am I invited to feel that I know how this client should live her/his life?
- By knowing so much, am I inviting my clients to take a stance of not knowing about themselves? Is this what I want to do? If I knew less, would they be invited to know more?
- Is my knowing about this case restraining me from gathering further information that might be useful? If I knew less, what other areas of inquiry might occur to me?

Editorial Guideline 9: Not Working Harder Than Clients

If the therapist is able to pay attention to the guidelines previously suggested, it is our experience that the ninth guideline will "automatically" be followed. An editorial position invites the client to be the author and to take the responsibility for that task; thus the client is working harder than the editor. It would be an unusual editor who would be willing to do all the writing and then give the client credit for it. It would also be an unusual client who would really feel like taking credit for work that he/she did not do.

Some Useful Questions for Therapists to Ask Themselves

- How has it come to be that I am more interested in the client's changing than the client is? How has it transpired that I care more about this client's life than she/he does?
- If I worked less, would the client be invited to work more?
- What dominant story in my past is suggesting that it is my job to work harder than the client? Where did that rule come from?

- How has "working harder" become synonymous with "helping better"? What if "working less hard" meant that I would be a better helper? What form would I want working less hard to take?

Case Dialogue Example

THERAPIST: I'm getting a bit uncomfortable here. It seems to me that I'm getting the message that what you are desiring is a miracle—for me to be able to make your life the way that it was. Is that at all accurate?

CLIENT: Well, actually, yes . . . I want you to make the terrible things that happened all right.

THERAPIST: Yeah, and I've been working real hard at that. I guess I'm beginning to get curious about what it is that you are willing to do in order to try to encourage that to happen.

CLIENT: I don't know what to do. That's why I'm here . . . I want you to tell me.

THERAPIST: So let's see if I understand. You want me to treat you as if you are not capable of doing any of this yourself? You'd rather me treat you as if you are incapable?

CLIENT: Well, not exactly. I just want you to tell me what to do.

THERAPIST: This our sixth session together, isn't it?

CLIENT: Yes, I believe so.

THERAPIST: In the previous five sessions, there where any number of times that I have made suggestions, and on a few occasions I've actually given you assignments. Do you remember any of those?

CLIENT: Yes . . . a few of them.

THERAPIST: And were any of those helpful to you?

CLIENT: No, somehow I just wasn't able to do any of them.

THERAPIST: So help me with my confusion. How is me telling you this time going to be any different?

CLIENT: I don't know.

THERAPIST: But somehow it still makes sense to you that what therapy is supposed to be about is for me to tell you to do something . . . and that somehow I will be able to come up with something that will make all the pain go away?

CLIENT: Yes . . . that's what I'd like, exactly.

THERAPIST: OK, I think I understand now. Let's say I told you to go home and come up with three things that you would be willing to do in order to help things be better in your life. Could you do that?

CLIENT: No, I'm not sure . . . it would be real hard!

THERAPIST: Yes, it probably would. But if that would help you start to feel better, would you want to do it?.

CLIENT: I don't know . . . I suppose, but I'm not sure I can.

THERAPIST: Yes, the old story would want you to believe that you can't. Why don't you give it a try anyway, and call me for another appointment when you've done it?

This represents an extreme example that was used with a client who was acting very helpless. We do not believe it was any coincidence, however, that after this conversation the client made some significant changes. It is our opinion that it interrupted an ongoing pattern of the therapist's working more and the client's working less.

Another Case Dialogue Example

THERAPIST: So you've decided that reading is just too hard for you, and that you're going to give up on being a reader?

CLIENT [an 11-year-old diagnosed as learning-disabled]: Yes, I've tried and tried, and I just can't do it!

THERAPIST: Yes, I understand that it is very difficult for you. You are very good at learning things that you can hear, but it's very hard for you to learn visually. I'll bet that really seems unfair to you at times.

CLIENT: Yes, it does. My brother doesn't have that problem at all.

THERAPIST: Yeah, I can see how that might even make it seem even more unfair.

CLIENT: Yeah.

THERAPIST: It seems that your parents have been working very hard to try and help you become a reader. Is that right?

CLIENT: Yes, they help me a lot . . . sometimes they also bug me a lot.

THERAPIST: I'm confused about something. Maybe you can help me. How is it that your parents care more about you being a reader than you do?

CLIENT: I don't know.

THERAPIST: It seems to me that they're willing to work very hard at it—even harder than you are. How did this happen?

CLIENT: I don't know.

THERAPIST: Do you agree that they do work harder at it than you do?

CLIENT: Yeah, I guess.

THERAPIST: Would it be OK if your parents accepted you as a nonreader? Would you want them to do that?

CLIENT: I don't know.

THERAPIST: Well, since they can both already read, and if it's OK with you to be a nonreader, would you like for them to accept that and not work so hard?

CLIENT: I don't know.

THERAPIST: Well, let's play with that idea a little bit. Let's say they did accept you as a nonreader, stopped bugging you about it, and loved you anyway. Let's say they were totally willing to do that. They were willing to read the menu for you in restaurants, take you to the bathroom so you didn't go in the wrong door—things like that—and of course accepted that you are going to flunk out of school because you can't read. If they accepted it completely and left it up to you, what would you want to do?

CLIENT: Uhmm . . . I'm not sure.

THERAPIST: Well, if you want to, why don't you think about it, and let your parents know what you would like to do—be a reader or a nonreader. And if you decide to be a reader, perhaps you could suggest to them how they could be the most helpful to you.

A couple of days later, this client requested a reading tutor. The parents made the child responsible for seeing that the appointments were kept, and explained that their job was paying for them. The child progressed very well in reading over the next 2 years, although it remained a difficult area.

Editorial Guideline 10:
Focusing on What Symptoms Depend Upon

Readers will remember that we conceptualize symptoms as part of a "wake-up call" that is inviting the client to consider a story re-vision. As such, symptoms are attached to an old story line rather than existing in isolation. We have found it useful to discover what parts of the story must continue to exist in order that the symptoms not change.

Some Useful Questions for Therapists to Ask Themselves

• What sort of standard are clients using to support the notion that they are not succeeding in life? What standard are they falling short of that is inviting them to story themselves as failures—and be depressed?

• If, instead of focusing on fear or anxiety (or any other symptom), I instead became curious about what fear depends on to stay strong, what would I find out? What sort of questions would I want to ask a client in this regard?

• How are things different for this client when the symptoms are not around? What does this difference suggest?

Case Dialogue Example

THERAPIST: So depression has been around for quite a while now—for several years. Can you help me understand how it has been able to stay strong for this length of time? What has it depended upon to accomplish that?

CLIENT [middle-aged female]: I'm not sure I know what you mean.

THERAPIST: Well, in my experience with other clients, it has seemed that much of the time depression has stayed strong by getting them to compare themselves to standards they feel they couldn't achieve, or to a situation they felt they couldn't change. I was wondering if it had done that with you.

CLIENT: For most of my adult life, I've been trying as hard as I can to be a good wife and mother. I don't know if that's what you mean or not.

THERAPIST: Have you succeeded at those tasks? And what does it mean to be a good wife and mother? How would you know if you had succeeded?

CLIENT: I've been a pretty good mother. My kids have turned out OK. As for the wife thing, I thought I was, but it doesn't appear to be so.

THERAPIST: And how do you know it isn't so?

CLIENT: The relationship is awful. I'm not even sure we like each other!

THERAPIST: And since it isn't good, that means you've failed as a wife?

CLIENT: It used to. Lately I've been coming to understand it may mean some other things as well. I've tried for years to change things, and it hasn't worked.

THERAPIST: Over all these years of trying, how much would you say that your own voice and preferences have been sacrificed?

CLIENT: Almost completely . . . however, I didn't know it at the time. It was just something that a woman did.

THERAPIST: And what prompted you to realize this was happening? It sounds like you received some sort of a call to change.

CLIENT: It was my children growing up, I think. Suddenly all that was left was the relationship that my husband and I didn't have.

THERAPIST: So it was OK to sacrifice your own preferences for your children, but when they left, things changed?

CLIENT: Yes. I realized just how much I had tried, and things still hadn't changed.

THERAPIST: So does depression depend upon that? Does it invite you to feel that your sacrifice was for nothing, and that you still have no right to your own preferences and desires?

CLIENT: Yes . . . and also that my husband doesn't care or understand. He doesn't feel the need for any change.

THERAPIST: And when you tell him how you feel?

CLIENT: He becomes angry and says it's ridiculous.

THERAPIST: So how much has depression relied upon the notion that the female voice is to be subordinate to the male voice . . . that your own preferences should not only go unattended, but that you don't even have the right to have them?

CLIENT: That's a big part of it. I am realizing that they are probably not going to be acknowledged or understood by my husband.

THERAPIST: And if they aren't validated by a male, does that mean they don't count?

CLIENT: Of course they count, but sometimes it seems they don't matter.

THERAPIST: So does depression try to remind you that you are losing your voice? Is that when it comes around?

CLIENT: Yes, it's stronger then.

THERAPIST: So depression seems to rely on some larger stories about males and females in order to stay strong. It tries to get you to believe that it will always be that way, and to feel guilty if you want it different. Is this accurate for you?

CLIENT: Yes, I would say that it is.

Editorial Guideline 11:
Asking "What Would It Mean" Questions

Guideline 11 can be illustrated in the case of a young adult female who was cooperating with the notion that she needed a man in order for her life to have meaning, and was experiencing sadness and depression as a result. The therapeutic dialogue went as follows:

THERAPIST: What would it mean if you don't find a steady boyfriend in the near future?

CLIENT: Well, I'll be alone all my life. I'll have no one. The older you get, the harder they are to find.

THERAPIST: Are there any other things that it would mean?

CLIENT: I could get so lonely and scared that I'll get into another abusive relationship and be unable to get out of it.

THERAPIST: Has this happened before?

CLIENT: Yes. I was in one for 5 years and almost never got out!

THERAPIST: So not having a boyfriend invites you to cooperate with a story that has an unhappy ending. It ends with you either being abused or alone.

CLIENT: Yeah, I guess so.

THERAPIST: No wonder you're feeling down. Those are pretty scary stories.

CLIENT: Yes, they are.

THERAPIST: So would your greatest fear be ending up alone, being abused, or something else?

CLIENT: Ending up all alone.

THERAPIST: And this fear suggests that you should have a boyfriend, even if he treats you badly?

CLIENT: Yes, but I don't want that either. I want someone who will respect me.

Editorial Guideline 12: Maintaining a Gender-Sensitive Stance

  Case Dialogue Example

The following case dialogue is representative of the type of processing that guideline 12 invites us to engage in with our clients. We feel that by not taking this area for granted, but rather by processing it, both the therapist and the client are invited to be aware of gender issues that may be influencing the session.

THERAPIST [male]: So you've had a long history of being dominated by the male voice . . . in fact, this domination has even taken the form of physical and sexual abuse on occasion. Is this correct?

CLIENT [female]: Yes. I grew up being afraid of men most of the time. I still am to some degree.

THERAPIST: This invites me to be very aware at this moment that I am male. Do you think this fact will influence the therapy in any way? Would you feel more comfortable with a female therapist?

CLIENT: I might feel more comfortable with a female, but I think that I need to work on being able to interact better with males, so in that regard it might be an advantage.

THERAPIST: So it might help you exercise your female voice in the presence of a male?

CLIENT: Yes, perhaps.

THERAPIST: When you are feeling dominated by the male voice, how is it that you would know? Are you able to tell?

CLIENT: Yes, usually . . . I get nervous and sort of jumpy in my stomach. I also become very quiet.

THERAPIST: If you started feeling that way in any of our sessions, would you be able to tell me? I would really appreciate it if you would. That way, I could stop doing whatever it is that is frightening to you that I might be unaware of.

CLIENT: Yes, I think I could tell you . . . one thing would be for you to keep your voice soft.

THERAPIST: So that would help insure that you didn't feel dominated, if I were able to speak in a very soft voice?

CLIENT: Yes, that would really help.

THERAPIST: I appreciate you letting me know that, and I will certainly try to do exactly that. If I forget, will you please remind me?

CLIENT: Yes.

Some Useful Questions for Therapists to Ask Themselves

• Do I come from a past that invites me to be gender-sensitive and mutual, or would the story I grew up in influence me otherwise?

• Do I honestly like the other gender, or if I am honest with myself, do I feel that my gender is superior?

• How much do the patriarchal notions of the culture I grew up in influence my view of the opposite gender? Are there ways in which I am under the spell of dominant cultural notions that I may have overlooked?

• Am I willing to learn about how to be a more effective therapist with the opposite gender, by letting therapists of that gender instruct me?

• Am I aware that males and females make different uses of languages in many instances? Would I be willing to alter my language in order to be a more effective therapist with the opposite gender?

• Am I consistently capable of maintaining a gender-neutral stance in therapist sessions, or do I inadvertently allow stereotypical views to influence me?

An Example of Gender Language Differences

Over the past year or so, we have been experimenting with using different language when discussing relationships with female clients. Feminist literature has suggested that females do not relate well to typically male language when discussing closeness or distance in relationships. Males, it seems, can tolerate and even relate to such phrases as "getting more distance between you and your parents," "divorcing yourself from your parents somewhat," "disconnecting from your family of origin so that you have more freedom," and the like. Females, however, seem to feel that such phrases imply that they must sever important ties. They relate better to language such as "reorganizing the relationship you have with your parents," "learning to care in ways that leave you less responsible," "realigning the relationship you have with your younger brother," and so on. We have found that using this type of language with our female clients has improved our effectiveness. This has invited us to wonder whether there are not many other instances where we use a "male language" and inadvertently miss connecting with our female clients. We would invite the reader to remember that the majority of the literature that has been used in teaching and training therapists has been authored by males. It is only very recently that the female voice has been given enough credence to be widely published. As a result, much of the language to which we have been exposed in our training has been male in its orientation. This is particularly accurate of medical-model language. Has the time come for the therapeutic community to develop a more gender-sensitive style of language?

The Reflecting Team as an Editorial Committee

Examples of Questions to Elicit the Hidden Text

• I have heard it said that anger is most often "hurt in disguise." Would you agree with that or not? How often would you say that anger depends on some underlying hurt for its expression?

• If you had expressed yourself when you were a child—if you had asked for what you needed—what do you imagine the response of others would have been? Would they have heard you and been able to respond, or would they have suggested that your feelings were somehow not valid?

• To what extent would you say that your cooperation with an angry lifestyle served to protect you as a child and adolescent? What did it protect you from?

• What would you say your greatest fear is? What is it that you would most wish to avoid?

Example of a Reflecting Team's Dialogue

TEAM MEMBER 1: I was struck with how much anger was discussed in the session. It seemed to me that anger exerts a very powerful hold on this family's life. I found myself wondering what anger primarily depends upon in order to stay so strong. What is it that would have to be dealt with in order for anger to grow weaker?

TEAM MEMBER 2: I think that's a very interesting question. In my experience, anger relies a lot on the perception of threat or harm. Is it possible that each of the members of the family feels threatened by the others, and the way they all protect themselves is with anger? I wonder what would happen if they spoke about their feelings of threat.

TEAM MEMBER 1: Or would it be more feelings of being hurt by the others?

TEAM MEMBER 3: That's what interests me the most. I've heard it said that about 95% of the time, anger is hurt in disguise. I wonder if anyone in the family would agree with that notion. Is the angriest member also the one who is feeling the most hurt and pain?

TEAM MEMBER 4: So if I'm following what you are saying, anger could be protecting them from discussing or dealing with other feelings: feelings which might be painful . . . feelings of being let down, or misunderstood, or attacked, or rejected . . . the list could go on and on. That's an interesting notion, that perhaps anger protects them from these sorts of things. I wonder if any of them would agree that anger helps them in some ways, while at the same time being destructive?

TEAM MEMBER 3: Yes, you heard what I was saying very accurately. Of course, I don't know if this seems accurate to the members of this family or not. Perhaps they could tell us.

Examples of Therapist Questions
Following the Reflecting Team's Stories

• Of the stories you just heard about you/your family, which of them appeals to you the most?
• Of the stories you just heard, which did you find the most accurate?
• Which of the team's accounts did you disagree with the most? Why?
• Where any of you surprised at anything that you heard? Did any of the stories invite you to realize anything about your family that you hadn't before?
• What would be necessary for you/your family to begin to live the story you like the most?

CHAPTER 5

Keeping the Story
Re-Vision Alive, Well,
and in Charge

Once a client is on her/his way in a story re-vision, it becomes the therapist/editor's job to encourage a continuation of this process. The new story, because of its relative recency, will remain vulnerable to subversion by the treachery of the old story, because of the powerful outside influences that authored this account initially. Old stories do not die easy deaths; in fact, our experience suggests that they do not die at all! Instead, they continue to extend invitations to the person throughout the remainder of her/his life. Our goal is not to do away with old stories so that they never tempt our clients again, but rather to acquaint people with optional story versions that they can use to regain control over their lives. In our thinking, the question is not whether old stories will exist and continue to entice clients, for we assume that they will; it is whether these outdated accounts will be in charge. Thus, it becomes very important that re-visions be given every opportunity to become strong, especially while in their infancy. This chapter focuses on methods and techniques that we have found useful in the maintenance of new stories. We continue to use Cindy's case (see Chapter 3) to illustrate how our approach can be applied over the entire course of therapy. The chapter concludes as Chapter 3 and 4 have done, with an appendix of suggestions, questions, and case dialogue examples; the appendix ends with an itemized summary of Cindy's case.

RECRUITING AN AUDIENCE
FOR THE NEW STORY

The best example of recruiting an audience for a new story that we have encountered is the Alcoholics Anonymous model of working with people under the influence of alcoholic lifestyles. It is possible to view the meetings of this organization as being centered around providing audiences that listen to, and validate, the stories of its members. This process involves the sharing of an old story, which could be entitled "Alcoholic," as well as that of a new story, which could be entitled "Sober." The efficacy of such validation and support should not be underestimated in the process of creating enduring change. Although new stories are very vulnerable to counterattack by old notions and outside influences, they become less so when they are validated by audiences or "witnesses." An excellent example is provided by the following case dialogue, in which a 9-year-old male shared his voice with those in attendance on just such a topic.

THERAPIST (*to parents*): I understand you feel there has been a relapse—that Johnny has let anger get the better of him again.

MOTHER: Yes, that's correct . . . we thought he was a lot better, but it seems that wasn't so. We're thinking that maybe all the change he made before was fake or something.

THERAPIST: I see. (*To the father*) And are you feeling that way too?

FATHER: Yeah, I suppose I am. He really blew it!

THERAPIST: So let me see if I understand. He was able to do his chores at home without anger taking him over, and this has stopped. Is that correct?

MOTHER: Well . . . no . . . he's still doing that.

THERAPIST: How about his homework? Have the temper tantrums revisited him there?

FATHER: No, he's still doing OK there too.

THERAPIST: Uhmm . . . I'm confused. How is it that he's relapsed?

FATHER: He hasn't. He's still doing well in those other areas. It's just that last night he really embarrassed us at a game. He yelled a profane word that I'd rather not say.

THERAPIST: Oh, I see. I understand how it is that you are so upset. However, I understood that anger had continued to get the better of him in sports . . . that sports is sort of anger's "last stand." I seem to remember you thinking that would probably be the hardest area for him to take control of. Is that right?

MOTHER: Yes, for sure. He just doesn't seem to be able to control himself when he doesn't do well in sports.

THERAPIST (*to child*): I'd like to congratulate you on your victories over anger so far. It's really good to hear that you are still able to do your chores and homework without it taking over. Can you help me understand what has to happen before you will be strong enough to do that in sports?

CHILD: Yeah, it's simple . . . I just need a few more victories in these other areas first . . . but I need people to notice. They don't count if people don't notice.

THERAPIST: Wow . . . let me see if I've got this. You're telling me that if others will give you credit for beating anger in other areas of your life, that some time in the future you will become strong enough to do it in sports too?

CHILD: Yes, that's correct.

THERAPIST: How would you like for other people to notice?

CHILD: For them to tell me that they saw me not getting angry.

THERAPIST: So Mom and Dad would have to be on the alert . . . and catch you not being angry in situations where you could have been. Is that it?

CHILD: Yeah, that would help.

THERAPIST: And if they do that, you think that you'll become stronger and stronger over time?

CLIENT: Yes.

THERAPIST: Isn't that interesting! He has the notion that he needs some more practice in the areas which are easier first, and that if he gets it, and if it gets noticed, he will be able to beat anger in areas where it has been in charge before. (*To the parents*) What do you think? Do you think it's worth a try?

FATHER: Yeah, it probably is. He has improved a lot over the last couple of months.

THERAPIST: Was the episode at the game able to get you to forget that?

MOTHER: I guess it did. It's really hard to remember when you're so embarrassed.

THERAPIST: Sure it is . . . really hard. How many times do you think you could catch him being not angry over the next week?

MOTHER: Oh . . . let me see, we'd really have to watch. Maybe 10 times.

THERAPIST: Wow, that's a lot! I was thinking more like three to five . . . do you think you could catch him five?

FATHER: If we paid attention, I'm sure we could.

THERAPIST: Sounds worth a try. Let me know how it goes.

Over the next week, the parents were able to "catch" their son not getting mad some 15 times! This trend continued, and 3 weeks later the son again had an occasion to let anger get the better of him at a sporting event. This time, however, he turned to his parents in the stands and gave them a wink. This major victory over anger led to an increasing ability on the son's part to control the influence of anger in his life.

Not only are new stories difficult for clients to maintain; they are also hard for other people to "trust." In the face of continuing evidence of trouble, it is very easy to forget that progress has been made, and to treat the identified clients as if they are no different at all. When therapists encounter outside audiences being dominated by an old story, it is very important to try to "catch these people up" with the new story, to supply an alternate audience that validates the new story, or both. Audiences that support and document change cannot be overemphasized. When other people validate, notice, and reinforce new stories, there is a strong invitation for the re-visions to survive. Often this will occur as a by-product of client change, giving the therapist a golden opportunity to punctuate such behaviors. In a recent case, a professional man, who had several females in his employ reported that he had arrived at the workplace to find a box of candy on his desk, with the following note attached:

"We don't know how you are making the changes that you are, but please keep it up!" The therapy with this client involved lessening the influence of anger in his life. Those he worked with had obviously noted his story re-vision, and had felt strongly enough about it to tell him. This event had a tremendous impact upon the client, and added an increased impetus to the survival of his new story.

In spite of the emergence of a story re-vision, however, the significant others in a client's life are sometimes so heavily under the influence of a problem-saturated past that they will be understandably restrained from noticing and validating the new story's existence. The continued presence of such restraint is usually reinforced by the fact that the old story seldom, if ever, dies a complete death, but rather is still partially in evidence in the identified client's life. Such a situation can stand as a major impediment to the survival of the re-vision. This can be illustrated by the reciprocal-invitation patterns therapists regularly encounter in cases involving adolescents highly influenced by underresponsibility, and parents caught up in a story of superresponsibility (see Chapter 3). In such instances, it is common to find that small movements on the part of the adolescents toward a story of increased responsibility are overlooked or discounted by parents and teachers. This invites the adolescents to cooperate with the notion that nothing they do will make a difference, and to engage in further behaviors that are viewed as irresponsible by others. Such a sequence can effectively stop, or at the very least detour, a story that is on the road to being re-visioned. We have been very interested in experimenting with techniques that keep significant others abreast of an identified client's new story, and thereby invite them to provide positive reinforcement for its continuation. Some techniques are described below.

1. Writing Letters to Significant Others

We have found that letters inviting others to "catch up" with the new stories being authored by our clients can be a very powerful adjunct to therapy (White & Epston, 1989). Such a letter can be written exclusively by a client or a therapist, or can be a joint venture involving them both. In any of these forms, the intent of the letter is to provide those who have been most affected by the old story with information that will invite a re-storying of the client. Often, for a variety of reasons, significant others will have not been in attendance during the therapy sessions, and thus will lack important information upon which a new view of the client can be based. Letters can bridge this gap by providing those who have not been present with such information. Examples of such letters can be found in the end-of-chapter appendix.

2. Conducting Interviews with Significant Others

When others are willing to come to the therapy, interviews can sometimes accomplish as much as, or more than, letters. Such interviews center around themes that emphasize the interconnectedness of people, and the invitational loops that can develop as a result. The following example is offered in this regard:

THERAPIST: Let me see if I understand. You have grown tired of your husband's [the client] lack of responsible behavior . . . you view him as just another child. That's the reason you encouraged him to come in for therapy?

CLIENT'S WIFE: Exactly. I already have three children, I don't need another one! He needs to grow up.

THERAPIST: What are some things he would do that he's not doing now, that you would view as signs he was growing up?

WIFE: He would take some responsibility for the finances, for paying the bills.

THERAPIST: Do you take care of all of that presently?

WIFE: Yes, it has always been that way at our house.

THERAPIST: If he was ready to assume some of that responsibility—let's say, something like sitting down and paying the bills at the first of the month—which would be harder: for him to do that, or for you to let him?

WIFE (*after long period of silence*): My goodness! I'm not sure . . . I don't think I could trust him to do that . . . it would never get done.

THERAPIST: So which would be harder: for him to change his story, or for you to believe that he could and give him the opportunity to do so?

WIFE: Uhmm . . . after all this time, it would probably be harder for me to believe that he could.

THERAPIST: So what would he have to do in order for you to believe that he can change, and that he is changing?

WIFE: Boy, that's a good question! I'm not sure there's anything he could do at this point in time.

THERAPIST: And would that be consistent with others in his life . . . his parents, too? Has anyone ever treated him like he had what it takes to grow up?

WIFE: Well, now that you mention it . . . no, I guess nobody has. His parents certainly haven't.

THERAPIST: Uhmm . . . it would have been difficult for him to have learned, wouldn't it?

WIFE: Yes, I guess it would.

THERAPIST: So if he decided to experiment with being more responsible, would you want to support this . . . to act as if he could?

This type of questioning emphasizes that stories are connected and do not develop in isolation. It invites significant others to entertain the notion that if they desire change in a member of their family system, it will be helpful if they can not only believe that the person can change, but notice it when he/she does. It invites them to view their role in the storying of the identified client.

3. Conducting Interviews with the Client

Clients are usually understandably excited about their re-visioned view of themselves, and expect and hope that others will share this excitement with them. As previously suggested, however, this is often not the case. Others are often afraid to trust that an identified client's altered behaviors will survive, and may even feel that they are being "set up" to be hurt and disappointed yet again. This can be very discouraging to the identified client, sometimes to the point of inviting her/him back into behaviors that are consistent with the old story. This, of course, only serves to reify the old story for everyone concerned. In an attempt to counteract such forces and influences, we have experimented with conducting sessions that "inoculate" the client against such disappointment, and (we hope) render it more likely that the new story will survive in the face of doubt and mistrust by others. The following case dialogue serves as an example of this process:

CLIENT: It doesn't seem to matter what I do. My teachers at school still treat me like I'm a troublemaker. They blame me for everything.

THERAPIST: It sounds like your teachers are having trouble catching up with your new story. It seems that their view of you is still influenced by the way things used to be.

CLIENT: Yeah, that's for sure! They don't know that I've changed.

THERAPIST: Either that, or they don't think that the changes will last. Do you think it's possible that they are afraid to trust that your new story is permanent?

CLIENT: Well, maybe, but that's not fair. They've been wanting me to be different all this time, and now that I am they don't treat me any differently.

THERAPIST: Does the old story ever try and use this to convince you to give up, to not care . . . to just go back to the old ways of being?

CLIENT: Yeah, sometimes it does . . . I mean, what's the use? They're never going to see me any differently.

THERAPIST: Uhmm . . . if the old story can get you to believe that, then it could regain control of your life, couldn't it? That sounds like a really good strategy for the old story to use . . . to try and convince you that if others don't notice your new story, you should give it up. Do you think that the old story will be able to succeed in this way?

CLIENT: I don't know. It's pretty discouraging at times. I try real hard, but nobody seems to notice.

THERAPIST: Yes, I can see where that would be really frustrating for you. It would be nice if others could give you credit for the changes that you've made and are making. But what if it takes them a while longer to do that? Will the old story be able to use that to stop your progress?

CLIENT: I don't want it to, but sometimes . . . I don't know.

THERAPIST: It occurs to me that if the old story could manage to convince you to give up, then your teachers would be sure that they were right . . . that the changes couldn't last. I wonder, are they right? Will the new story fade away, or will you prove them wrong? I wonder how long you'd have to hang in there before they started to realize that you've changed?

CLIENT: I don't know. I'm not sure I could convince them if I did it forever!

THERAPIST: Well, the old story would really be pleased if it could get you to believe that! What would your new story have to say?

CLIENT: It would say that I should hang in there . . . that if I try long enough, they will have to notice.

THERAPIST: Uhmm . . . that's quite a different-sounding story. Which of those stories would you prefer to believe?

CLIENT: I'd like to believe the second one, but it's hard sometimes.

THERAPIST: Of course it is . . . it's real hard and frustrating. Do you think that you want to go for it anyway, or do you want to let the old story win and prove your teachers right?

CLIENT: No, I don't want them to be right.

THERAPIST: Well, I'm with you! I think it would be great fun to prove them wrong. I'd love to see you do it. Of course, in order to do that, you might have to somewhat ignore others' stories about you. Do you feel up to that?

CLIENT: I'm willing to try it a while longer . . . and see what happens.

THERAPIST: Maybe we should explore that a little. What sort of things could you do that would really invite them to side with a new story about you?

CLIENT: Uhmm . . . I don't know. It seems nothing will do it.

THERAPIST: For sure, that's the way it would seem in the old story . . . the old story would want you to believe that. But despite that feeling, can you think of anything that would really get their attention?

CLIENT: Well . . . if I started making better grades, that might help.

THERAPIST: Is making better grades something that is in line with your new story? Is that something you would like to do?

CLIENT: A little better . . . maybe not as much as my parents would want, but a little better.

THERAPIST: So if you began to improve your grades to the extent that you would like to, you think that your teachers would be invited to revise their story about you somewhat.

CLIENT: Yeah, probably.

THERAPIST: Do you think that's worth a try?

CLIENT: Yeah, maybe . . . I'll think about it.

In Cindy's case, several sessions of this type were held to try to insure the survival of her new story. The aim of such sessions was to address issues regarding her family members' reaction to her new story, as well as to wonder whether the old story might use their lack of understanding and support as a means of regaining lost territory in her life. The process was much the same as that outlined in the example above, with questions being posed in the following areas:

• If the old story wanted to regain control, would it be likely to counterattack via using her family's opinions?
• If the old story were able to succeed in such an endeavor, what would it be able to get her to think and do?
• Did she think she would be able to continue her new story even if her family never became able to validate it? Or would this render it impossible for her to continue?
• What sorts of behaviors on her part would invite the members of her family to entertain the notion that they had been incorrect about her? What sorts of behaviors would influence them to believe that they had been correct?

4. Using a Reflecting Team as an Audience

A reflecting team can also be utilized in this process of recruiting an audience that will notice and reinforce the existence of a new story. Quite often, we schedule sessions with a reflecting team in attendance, so that the client can relate his/her story in the presence of an attentive and appreciative audience. An interview that consistently compares the client's old story with that of the new story offers ample potential for team reflections that applaud and validate the new story, as well as the process used to accomplish such changes. Examples of such comparison questions can be found in the appendix. (Chapter 4 has provided a more thorough discussion of the reflecting team's functioning.)

In Cindy's case, as previously mentioned in Chapter 3, a reflecting team was used in connection with the ritual burning of the specifications cards that she had determined had no place in her new story. This was done to provide a larger audience that could validate the step she was taking. A brief excerpt from the team's reflections is provided in the appendix.

USING LETTERS TO CONSOLIDATE NEW STORY ROLES

Using letters as an adjunct to the counseling process has seemed to us to be a natural outgrowth of doing therapy from a narrative stance. Stories take on added meaning and permanence when they are written down. They can be re-examined, changed, and edited. The use of the written word seems to render them "more real" and open to analysis. Readers interested in an in-depth discussion of how the written word can be employed therapeutically are referred to White and Epston (1989). In this work the authors outline the basis of the narrative analogy, as well as giving examples of various types of therapeutic letters: letters of invitation, letters of prediction, letters of reference, letters for special occasions, letters as narrative, and self-story letters.

In our practice, we have been interested in the use of letters for the following purposes:

1. To insure that we have heard our clients' stories accurately. Letters give a client the opportunity to "edit the editor."

2. To give ourselves time to ponder cases outside of the rapid-fire atmosphere of therapeutic conversation. We have found that many good ideas occur to us after interviews have ended. Letters to the clients provide the opportunity to utilize these ideas without waiting for the next session.

3. To "extend" the effect of the therapy sessions, and render it less likely that a client will "forget" the conversation. Our clients have told us that the letters help them remember what transpired in sessions, as well as giving them something to refer to on a regular basis if they so desire.

4. To render a new story more "newsworthy" by documenting the various exceptions to the old story that surfaced during an interview.

5. To provide a written "double description" for a client that contrasts the old story with the new story.

6. To expand upon the therapist/client relationship. We have found that clients are very appreciative of the time and effort that letter writing requires of a therapist.

In our experience, such letters provide a very powerful tool for reifying a new story, and for rendering it less likely to fall prey to the counterattacks of the old story and its hidden text. Examples of letters we have written to our clients can be found in the end-of-chapter appendix, including one that was written to Cindy after a session held during the early stages of her therapy.

STAYING BEHIND THE CLIENT

In order for behaviors and thoughts that fall outside the influence of the old story to be considered important, they must somehow be rendered valid and sufficient by everyone concerned. Conversely, if those involved treat such unique thoughts and behaviors as if they are insignificant, or not of sufficient volume or duration, it is likely that they will be discounted. One way in which thoughts and behaviors that can be utilized as part of a new story can be inadvertently rendered invalid is for the client and significant others to "jump ahead," rather than being pleased with what has occurred. We use the word "inadvertently" because we believe that most people jump ahead because they think it is helpful, and not because they are trying to make sure that change is retarded.

One of us (Doan) recently had an experience that illustrates this point. While on the golf course, Doan had finally figured out a way to improve his putting stroke, and as a result had improved his score significantly (from 92 to 86). A friend who was playing in the same group said very casually, "I'll bet it will be no time until you are shooting even par.'' Suddenly the 86 seemed tarnished and dull, when only moments before it had seemed cause for some sort of celebration. This jumping ahead, no matter how well intentioned, had emphasized what Doan had not been able to do (shoot par) instead of what he had done (improve by six strokes). If instead, the comment had been "Wow, 86! I can't believe you were able to improve by six strokes in one round," the meaning constructed would probably have been quite different.

This is a very simple but powerful way of reinforcing new stories so that they have a greater chance of survival. We are again indebted to Michael White (1989) for this information. Stated simply, this notion suggests that the therapist can be of more help to a client by ''staying behind'' the new story than by ''jumping ahead'' of it. It results in emphasizing what the client has done, instead of calling attention to what remains to be accomplished. This can be further illustrated by comparing two possible conversations between a parent and a fifth-grade child.

Conversation 1

PARENT: I see that you got a 75 on your spelling paper last week in school.

CHILD: Yes.

PARENT: You can do much better than that. I expect you to make at least an 85 on all of your school work. Anything less than that is unacceptable.

CHILD: I did the best I could.

PARENT: Did you study?

CHILD: Yes.

PARENT: Evidently not enough. You will study for an hour every day after school until your get your score up to 85. Is that understood?

Conversation 2

PARENT: I see you made 75 on your spelling paper last week.

CHILD: Yes.

PARENT: That means that you got 75 out of 100 correct! What did you do in order to accomplish that?

CHILD: I studied some.

PARENT: Really? You think that helped you get 75 right?

CHILD: Yes.

PARENT: Well, you certainly got a lot more of them right than you did wrong. What was the difference between the ones you got right and the ones you got wrong?

CHILD: The ones I got wrong were harder words. They were longer. I didn't even know what a couple of them meant.

PARENT: So the ones you got right were words you understood the meaning of . . . and had fewer letters in them.

CHILD: Yes.

PARENT: Would you want to make a higher score, or is 75 OK with you?

CHILD: I wouldn't mind it being a little higher.

PARENT: What would you need to do to raise it if you wanted to?

CHILD: Study a little more . . . and maybe ask you what some of the words meant . . . the ones I didn't understand.

PARENT: You know, I think you're right . . . that would probably work. Would you want to do that next time?

CHILD: Yes, probably.

This is a very similar concept to the old question ''Is the glass half empty or half full?'' We have found that emphasizing the full portion often results in more water being added to the glass, whereas focusing on the empty portion results in even more water somehow evaporating.

RE-VISIONING CLIENTS AS EXPERTS
ON THEIR OWN STORIES

As clients gain in the ability to exercise their voices in the author-ship of the stories they call their lives, we are very interested in providing invitations to continue this process. Initially, our intent is to provide yet another aid in the survival of these new stories, but later, as clients become even more skilled and capable, they can also provide a great service to other people and organizations. Clients who are successfully involved in the process of story re-vision have wonderful tales to tell. Their narratives are about overcoming the odds, defeating demons and dragons, and going on daring quests and adventures; heroes and heroines are the central characters. Providing them with the opportunity to tell their tales can be a very powerful adjunct to their therapy, as well as being an empowering force in the lives of those who are privileged to hear them. We have used the following techniques to accomplish this end.

1. Making Videotapes of Clients

Some time ago, a partner of Doan's suggested that it would be interesting to have a library of videotapes documenting the changes accomplished by successful clients (Mitchell, personal communication, 1991). It was his notion that such tapes not only would be a very powerful experience for the therapists and clients, but could also be used with other clients to good effect. Since that time, we have had several opportunities to experiment with this process, and our experience has been positive enough to recommend it to the reader.

The basic idea is to invite clients to see themselves as experts on changing their stories—experts with ideas that will be potentially valuable to others. Such a tape accomplishes several purposes:

1. It provides the client with yet another opportunity to tell her/his story and have it listened to with respect.

2. It provides the therapist with the chance to get an account that compares the new story with the old story across time, thus rendering distinctions between the two very clear.

3. It invites the client to "perform meaning" about herself/himself as a person who has some expertise in what it takes to re-vision a story.

4. It documents and preserves this for the client to keep and refer to later.

5. It provides the therapist with a resource that he/she can use with other clients who are in similar circumstances.

6. It provides a forum for the therapist, client, and others to learn what some potential ingredients for successful change might be.

We have found this a very powerful and useful tool, and are thankful that modern technology has given us the opportunity to film our clients "in the act" of living their story re-visions. The end-of-chapter appendix contains a partial transcript of such a session.

2. Arranging for Clients to Speak to Groups

Arranging for clients to speak to groups accomplishes many of the outcomes listed above, with the exception of preserving the experience on tape (although this can be done as well). Doan has made use of his position as a university instructor to accomplish this purpose. Some of his clients have been willing to come and speak to classes of graduate students, and share the process of their story revision with them. The same can be done with almost any group of people who might be interested in hearing a story about successful change and re-vision. The added advantage of this process is that it provides a live audience for the story, which further validates the journey a client has made.

3. Utilizing Clients in Therapy Sessions for Others

It is also possible to promote former clients to the status of "consultants," and to use their expertise in helping other clients in actual therapy sessions. Recently, two female clients/consultants were invited to share their story with another female who was just beginning the therapy process. The new client had been in several types of therapy, and was very skeptical about the potential of "yet another round" in the easing of the tyranny of depression in her life. In answer to her question "Do you really think this can do any good?", the therapist suggested that she visit with two women who had also experienced the oppressive influence of depression, and ask them the same question. She agreed, and the session was arranged. In looking back, it would be difficult to determine which party received the most from the conversation that ensued—the therapist, the new client, or the consultants. Suffice it to say that the experience seemed to play an important role in the successful departure from a depressed lifestyle on the part of the new client; it is probable that it also strongly invited the two consultants to continue their new stories. As for the therapist, he was influenced to schedule such sessions more often.

Cindy was one of the female consultants referred to above. She readily accepted the invitation to be so involved, and very succinctly shared the story of her change journey with the new client. The therapist simply asked her to share the portions of her story that she thought would be most helpful, and invited the new client to ask questions. This provided her with yet another opportunity to reify her new story by telling it one more time.

CONCLUDING COMMENT

New stories do not survive automatically; if they do survive, they are not always given the credit or validation required for them to make a significant difference in clients' view of themselves. It is often necessary to render the details and characteristics of new stories so visible that both the clients and significant others will be aware of their existence. This is an important process in maintaining behaviors and ideas that will lead to lasting change. The only stories that count are ones that people are sufficiently aware of to recite into being. This chapter has outlined several methods for inviting both clients and others into recitations that emphasize resources and strengths, rather than versions that fall prey to the problem-saturated narratives of old stories.

APPENDIX: THERAPEUTIC EXAMPLES

Recruiting an Audience for the New Story

1. Writing Letters to Significant Others

The following is an example of the type of letter we have written to significant others in an attempt to catch them up with the new story of a client. It has been altered in order to protect the confidentiality of those involved.

Dear Parents,

Congratulations on your great escape from the clutches of family trouble and conflict. Your son reports that it has now been a month since any significant conflict or fighting has occurred! You should all feel very proud of this accomplishment. As for me, I am somewhat amazed by this progress. I expected, from knowing your family, that you would make strides against trouble, but never did I imagine that it would occur to such an extent so quickly. Again, congratulations!

The purpose of this letter is much like the last one I sent you: to "catch you up" on the work that your son and I have been doing together. I felt it especially important to do so because of our last session—a session in which he continued to surprise me with the depth of his maturity and thoughtfulness. I went into the session on the watch for trouble, and once again found more evidence of victories over trouble than I did defeats. He keeps catching me somewhat off guard. At any rate, at some point in the session I asked him whether he thought the two of you knew some of the things about him that were emerging. He said he was pretty sure that you were unaware of most of them. I wondered whether knowing them would be helpful to you or not, and he thought that it would. So, here is a letter from both of us to let you in on some of his thoughts, feelings, and desires, in the hope that you will find them both interesting and useful. In the interest of simplicity, we have listed them below:

1. He is somewhat "allergic" to praise. It is very hard for him to take because he has the feeling he really doesn't deserve it at times. This allergy influences him not to respond to praise; in fact, he usually ignores it. He thinks this might give people the idea that he doesn't appreciate it, when actually it's just that he has this allergy.

2. He believes in a higher power that stands for good, and an opposing power that stands for bad. His conceptualization of this higher power is quite advanced, in that it is not human at all, but is far beyond that—so much so that we probably cannot even imagine it.

3. He thinks that we humans sort of "stand at the crossroads" in terms of which of these powers will hold sway. He places the odds at 50–50 that we will opt for good. He realizes that this choice exists for him as well, and he is determined to decide on his own. In fact, he says that when people try to force him to choose either way, it only renders him less inclined to go in the direction they are recommending.

4. When he is older (20), he plans to be even more mature than he is now, to have a more informed view of life, and to be in college (in some other state, he hopes, so he can get "two types of education at once").

5. He thinks that it would be nice to be in love by age 20, but that it isn't the top priority. He thinks that he can be a very complete person in

his own right, and doesn't "need a woman" in order to be emotionally OK. (I was really impressed with this one, and can only hope I can get my 10-year-old son to feel as good about himself.)

6. He spends lots of time alone, especially in his room, because "life happens so quickly, and if you aren't careful it will pass right by. You need to stop and pay attention to it regularly." His time alone is mostly spent thinking about life, pondering what he wants out of it, and asking himself questions concerning it. When he is alone, he can do this without others diverting his thoughts.

After hearing all this, I was hardly able to convince myself that your son is the tender age that he is; it invited me to view him as much older. I asked him if that was ever a problem for him—if people expected him to grow up faster than he was able, to treat him as if he was older than he is. He said that at times he felt this way, but that it was his job to grow up, and that he is determined to do so! I wish I could "bottle" this attitude so some of my other adolescent clients could drink it!

It occurs to me that the two of you must certainly be doing many things right as parents to produce such a thoughtful, intelligent young man. I hope you can appreciate the job you've done. We hope that this letter is just the beginning of a story in which you feel that you are competent parents who needn't worry so much about your parenting skills. If you sided with such a notion, one can only wonder how the next chapter in your "parenting novel" might read!

Respectfully,

Your son and his therapist

2. Conducting Interviews with Significant Others

Provided below is a sampling of questions which we have found useful in conducting interviews to try to sensitize significant others to changes in the identified client.

• Which would be harder: for your son to change his story, or for you to notice and give him credit if he did?

• How much of a change would be necessary before you felt safe to notice and give your sibling credit for it?

• In the event that your daughter is changing, and somehow you don't notice it, what effect would you think that would have on her?

• Is it possible that small changes have already occurred in your spouse's story, but that the trouble of the past has restrained you from seeing it?

• How many positive behaviors can be erased by one episode of trouble?

• Is it possible that one way in which trouble has taken over your family is to get everyone to ignore good things when they happen, but to be hypervigilant concerning problems?

• Do you think that change usually occurs in big, miraculous ways, or in small, progressive steps? If it was occurring in small, progressive steps in your family, would that be OK, or would it be discounted?

3. Conducting Interviews with the Client

Here is a sampling of questions that can be used to try to inoculate clients against counterattacks by the old story, based upon others' not validating their new story.

• What sort of behaviors invite others to maintain their old story about you? Do you think you are currently doing anything that would tend to insure that they continue to view you in the same old way?

• What could you do that would invite others to understand that you are living a new story these days? Can you think of things you could do that would be almost impossible for them to overlook?

• What would be a reasonable amount of time to give others to realize that you are very serious about authoring a new story for yourself? Do you think they should recognize it immediately, or do you think it's more likely it will take them a while to catch up with you?

• Which would be harder: for others to give you credit for small changes, or for you to give credit to them? Is it possible that you are overlooking small changes in the way they view you, in much the same way they are overlooking things in you?

• Which has the more powerful influence in your current story: your opinion of yourself, or others' opinions of you? How much are you able to validate yourself, and how much do you rely on others to validate you?

• If others' view of you changed slowly over time—if they caught up with your story slowly but surely—would that be OK? Or do you expect them to catch up suddenly and all at once? If they could only change slowly, could you accept that? Would you want them to accept that in you?

4. Using a Reflecting Team as an Audience

Some Useful Questions

The following is a representative list of therapeutic questions that can be used to provide a reflecting team with information concerning a client's "journey." These questions focus on differences and changes that have occurred across time, giving the client the opportunity to story this process in the presence of an audience whose members will give him/her feedback at the end of the session.

• What would the team need to know in order to understand how things were in your old story? What would you want to share with them in this regard?

• How are things different for you now? How has the story changed?

• On a scale from 0 to 10, where would you rate yourself when you first came in for counseling, and where would you rate yourself now?

• What would you title your old story? What is your current story's title?

• How do you account for these changes? What have you done to accomplish this result?

• If you were going to advise the team on how to work with clients such as yourself, what would be most important for them to know?

• What do you think your story means to the team? What sort of things do you imagine they might be thinking as they listen?

Case Dialogue Example

Following is an excerpt of the reflecting team's dialogue from the transcript of the session in which Cindy burned her specification-of-personhood cards (see Chapter 3). This serves as an example of using the reflecting team as an appreciative and validating audience. Once again, the example is not as pertinent as it might be if the reader had been able to hear the session that preceded the reflections. In spite of this, however, we hope that it gives the reader an idea of the types of reflections used in this process.

TEAM MEMBER 1: I'm real impressed with the amount of insight Cindy has developed in relationship to the rules which were running her life. She really seemed to have a grasp on what she was doing and why. I found myself wondering if she is aware of just how far she has come in this regard. Does she give herself credit for it?

TEAM MEMBER 2: Yeah. If you had just walked in and heard all of the things she has realized, you might conclude that these had just recently occurred. But to find that she has been working on this for such a long time . . . why, it goes back several years to when she realized that she could change the hand in which she held the soap in the shower!

TEAM MEMBER 3: That was so impressive for me! That she could be aware of such a small change, and use it to accomplish other changes. I found myself wondering how she managed that. What steps were necessary for her to be so aware, and to use this in many other areas of her life?

TEAM MEMBER 2: Yeah, I may have trouble taking a shower tomorrow in my same old way *(laughing)*!

TEAM MEMBER 3: I know, I'll have to start putting my panty hose on differently. It will never be the same again *(laughing)*!

TEAM MEMBER 2: I've considered beginning some of the changes I want to make in my life by putting my pants on differently each morning. Maybe there's something I can learn from her.

TEAM MEMBER 1: It was personally inspiring for me to see her burn those cards. Especially the one about making A's in graduate school all the time. I found myself cheering her on back here . . . saying, "Burn it, burn it, burn that sucker!"

TEAM MEMBER 4: That one really got to me. I found myself wondering if I could burn that card in my own life . . . I don't know if I could. In listening to her I could tell how much of a history these rules had for her—and for her sister, who seemed to identify with most of them. They came from a long time in the past. How did she manage to take back the control of her life from them? That must have been very hard to do. I'd like to hear more about exactly how she managed it.

TEAM MEMBER 3: I found myself wondering if the same sort of specifications existed in her mother's life as well,

TEAM MEMBER 1: Yeah, breaking old family patterns has been the hardest thing for me to do personally. I too would like to know how she has done this.

TEAM MEMBER 2: So maybe those rules have a real long history. I wonder how long they've been in her family?

TEAM MEMBER 3: Yes, it seemed that they've had a stranglehold on her much of her life . . . but now she's turning the tables on them. I have several clients trying to do the same thing. I wonder if she would be willing to act as a consultant for me in those cases?

TEAM MEMBER 1: Yeah, I agree . . . especially about the specifications which isolated her. They seem to have been particularly strong.

TEAM MEMBER 2: Yes, I remember her saying that while she was writing these cards that she felt like she was behind a brick wall. I was wondering, now that she's gone through the process of burning these specifications, what does she feel like now? Has part of the wall been torn down? Does she feel released?

TEAM MEMBER 4: One of the specifications I was particularly excited about her burning was that a woman should wait for others to read her mind, that they should be able to do that. Today is evidence that she has escaped that specification. By letting us in on this process, she stepped out of that rule. She didn't make us read her mind; she let us see it very clearly. She was so open that we didn't have to wonder or guess. I wonder if she realized that about today . . . that it really broke a lot of these rules?

TEAM MEMBER 1: Yeah, today was really the opposite of stopping growth. It was growth-producing . . . for all of us. I wonder if she realizes how much those of us behind the mirror have been touched and changed by what she did?''

Using Letters to Consolidate New Story Roles

The following are examples of the types of letters we have used in the effort to consolidate new stories, and to render them more impervious to counterattacks by the old story and the hidden text. Again, they have been altered to protect clients' confidentiality.

Example Letter 1

Dear Jane Doe,

Just a note to document our last session together. There were so many noteworthy items that it seemed only proper to preserve them in writing. So I thought I would send you a listing of the following ''newsworthy'' events.

1. It has been noted that in spite of many invitations to the contrary, you decided to return to work last Monday—and continued to go the remainder of the week! This seems evidence of a remarkable bit of reclaiming your life from the forces of depression and self-depreciation.

2. It also was noted that you left work early one day last week; in fact, you took the entire afternoon off! Thus, not only did you manage to turn the tables on depression and self-depreciation, but you also escaped from

the clutches of their foremost ally, perfectionism. This is particularly noteworthy in that it marks the first time you have left work to do something you wanted to do. In the past, the only thing that could get you to miss work and take a rest was depression.

3. You also reported that you have decided that you have too many "deadlines" in your life, and that their presence is impoverishing. This is quite different from the old story, which suggested that unless you had tons of deadlines you would amount to nothing.

4. As if this wasn't enough, you also have started to keep track of the rules and specifications that perfectionism uses to keep you in line. You have even written some of these down.

Thus, it seems that a new story is emerging—a story that is being based on premises quite different from those of the past. Please let me know whether you agree with this account, and feel free to alter it in any way that will be more accurate for your story.

Example Letter 2

Dear John Doe,

Here is my attempt at documenting your movement toward the revised person you have indicated you wish to become. Please feel free to edit or change this account in order that it might be more accurate from your point of view.

It seems that your friends have started to notice some changes in you. Specifically, they are beginning to become aware that anger is much less able to influence you than in the past. Proof of this can be found in the fact that you are getting many more social invitations to do things with your friends, and colleagues at work have started to comment on the changes. It seems that you are inviting others to revise their stories concerning you.

Accompanying this new view of others, it has been noticed that you are less defensive, less critical, and less caustic. This is line with your report that "I feel completely different," and that "anger is less automatic, and even when it comes around it doesn't stay as long."

I can't help wondering what this knowledge that others are seeing and validating your efforts at escaping anger means to you. What does this suggest about you as a person, and how do you account for your ability to accomplish these changes? Perhaps you can share this with me at our next session.

Example Letter 3

Dear Cindy,

I am sending you this letter to document our time together. I hope that you find it both interesting and useful.

You have a very interesting story. It has all the ingredients of a great novel. What an interesting cast of characters! Your story would have the theme of family tradition dominating the characters to a large extent, within an overarching aura of religion. It would also be the story of a family whose members are very much involved with one another, even to this very day. It is a story of family members with secrets, who in spite of their involvement leave *many things* unsaid. It would be about a family that has passed along a heritage of unsureness and doubt, mixed with a very rigid, all-or-nothing view of the world. It is certainly easy to understand how someone raised within such a story would get caught up in it, and be readily influenced by anger and confusion. It would be easy to feel as if one's character had been written almost entirely by other people—and to feel guilty when one tried to pick up the pen and write the story for oneself.

However, in spite of this tradition, you have not been completely overwhelmed. Instead, you have escaped from it in a number of ways. It seems you have experienced a wake-up call that has invited you out of a story titled "Passive Victim" and into a story titled "Happy Adult." Some of the indications of this wake-up call are the following:

1. Becoming more assertive (rather than aggressive)
2. Exercising each day
3. Being more selective of friends
4. Doing good things for yourself each day
5. Recognizing that you are a good teacher

It seems that you have already begun the process of authoring a new story for yourself. I will wait with curiosity as your story unfolds.

Staying Behind the Client

Several examples of the process of "staying behind" the client, as opposed to "jumping ahead," are included in the body of the chapter. The following example is also provided.

THERAPIST: So one of the things that the depressed lifestyle seems to depend on is an ongoing fear of interacting with women. Is that accurate?

CLIENT [middle-aged male]: Yes, I'm scared to death of talking to women.

THERAPIST: Is there any type of interaction with females that you could imagine yourself doing . . . you know, if you wanted to prove to fear that it wasn't going to have its way with you totally?

CLIENT (*after a long pause*): I might be able to ask a female for the time of day.

THERAPIST: Really? You think that you could overcome fear enough to ask a woman what time it is?

CLIENT: Yeah, I wouldn't want to, but I probably could.

THERAPIST: How many women during the next week could you ask?

CLIENT: Maybe 10.

THERAPIST: Wow, that sounds like a lot to me! I was thinking more like three or so. Would you want to try that?

CLIENT: Yes, I'll do my best.

Staying behind clients also involves framing success as somewhat less than the standard that they might set for themselves. In this particular case, the client managed to ask five women for the time during the subsequent week, and found himself involved in a short conversation with three of them. Although this sounds like a trivial occurrence for most of us, it was very meaningful for the client. It provided a unique outcome that could be used in a continuing process of story re-vision. The therapist followed up the client's report in the manner outlined in Chapter 3 (unique outcomes, unique accounts, unique redescriptions, and unique possibilities).

Re-Visioning Clients as Experts on Their Own Stories

1. Making Videotapes of Clients

The following dialogue was taken from an actual tape made with a client by Doan. Space limitations render it impossible to include the entire transcript of the conversation, but we hope that the following excerpt provides the reader with an adequate example of this process.

THERAPIST: I want to thank you for being brave enough to do this. Hopefully some other people will benefit from it. So let me start by formally stating, for those who might eventually watch this tape, that I have asked you to share your journey so others who are on similar trips can profit from your experience. I'll just ask you some questions about that process. Can we get a little bit of a feel for where you were when we started versus where you are now? When we first began, what sort of story were you caught up in?

CLIENT: I was being dominated by feeling responsible for everything that happened. I had to be too perfect . . . overperfectionism.

THERAPIST: So when we began, overresponsibility and overperfectionism were in charge, and despite us talking about any number of things which had influenced your story, you weren't able to separate those from your own self-picture.

CLIENT: Yes, I felt I was responsible because I'd gotten involved with those things.

THERAPIST: And it didn't matter what age you had been when these things happened . . . you were still responsible.

CLIENT: Yes, it didn't matter. I needed to be perfect and I wasn't.

THERAPIST: And when you weren't, what feelings did that invite?

CLIENT: Low self-esteem. Feelings that people didn't care for me because I wasn't measuring up.

THERAPIST: How much of your story was being dominated by perfectionism, overresponsibility, and self-depreciation back then?

CLIENT: I'd say from 90% to 95%.

THERAPIST: As I recall, you were also very much under the influence of depression.

CLIENT (*laughing*): Yes, that's for sure! I didn't feel good about anything.

THERAPIST: And the more you tried to be perfect, the more depression was able to weasel its way in . . . is that accurate?

CLIENT: Yes, that's very accurate.

THERAPIST: So how were you able to give these things the slip? What did you do to manage that?

CLIENT: I wrote down the rules I lived by, and began to ask myself which ones were good for me.

THERAPIST: So you went through a process of analyzing the rules that perfectionism and depression used to stay strong, and began to realize that all of them weren't your cup of tea?

CLIENT: Yes.

THERAPIST: Did you also began to realize you hadn't authored many of these rules?

CLIENT: Yes, and that I wasn't responsible for most of them.

THERAPIST: Was that helpful, this realization?

CLIENT: It wasn't at first because I didn't believe it . . . but when I started believing, it was very helpful.

THERAPIST: Do you remember what happened to start you believing that you weren't totally responsible?

CLIENT: I think it was realizing I could do positive things, like my hobbies, and that what others thought wasn't that important.

THERAPIST: So, there started to be glimpses that there were some things OK about you, as well as the realization that the things that weren't OK weren't totally being based upon your own rules.

CLIENT: Yes.

THERAPIST: Were you able to completely grasp this new view of yourself, or did it come and go?

CLIENT (*laughing*): No, it came and went!

THERAPIST: Can you remember coming in to see me thinking that you had totally relapsed . . . were back to ground zero?

CLIENT: Yes . . . but that's part of change. You have to realize that you can't give up if you want to change.

THERAPIST: Along about that time, we started talking about two stories, if I remember correctly. The old story, the one about a villainess—and the new story, the one about a heroine. Is that how you remember it?

CLIENT: Yes, that's accurate.

THERAPIST: You seemed to be able to relate to that. Especially the old story, that since you couldn't be perfect . . .

CLIENT: Since I couldn't be perfect, I had to be bad.

THERAPIST: And how about the new story, the one about the heroine that I saw you being?

CLIENT: I couldn't relate to that one at first. I couldn't vision it.

THERAPIST: But in spite of that, you decided that it fit you better than the other one.

CLIENT: Yes.

THERAPIST: How did you began doing that?

CLIENT: By thinking differently—being more positive. By getting rid of certain rules and adding others . . . and by congratulating myself for each small victory I achieved.

THERAPIST: So for the people who will watch this tape, what would you think would be most important for them to know?

CLIENT: To be kind to themselves, to realize that change is a process, and to give themselves credit for doing small things differently. To not try and change too fast, but to give it time.

2–3. *Arranging for Clients to Speak to Groups; Utilizing Clients in Therapy Sessions for Others*

The following are examples of the types of questions the therapist can use in order to facilitate clients' speaking to groups or to other clients:

• Could you give the audience a brief description of your old story and how it was influencing your life?
• How are things different for you now? How is your new story different from the old?
• How do you account for this change? What did you do that allowed you to begin authoring a different story for yourself?
• Is the old story entirely gone, or does it still try and influence you from time to time? How do you manage to hold it off?
• What was the first thing you managed to do that you identified as part of a new story for yourself?
• What would be the most important thing for people who are wanting a new story for themselves to realize or know? If you could only give them one piece of advice, what would it be?
• Did the old story give up easily, or did it counterattack several times?

An Overview and Summary of Cindy's Case

In order to give the reader a more coherent view of Cindy's case, we provide the following overview and summary. Please note that the processes of deconstruction and story re-vision were not completely separate; rather, they occurred simultaneously, with attention shifting between the two as seemed useful.

The Deconstruction Process

1. Interviewing and questioning Cindy so as to give her the space and opportunity to tell *her* story based upon *her* experience. To accomplish this the therapist paid close attention to the editorial guidelines discussed in Chapter 4.
2. Identifying and challenging the specifications that the old story relied on to stay strong. This was primarily done in three ways:

3. Externalizing the old story and its foremost ally, perfectionism.

4. Encouraging Cindy to write the specifications of the old story on separate 3 × 5 cards, and to sort these into stacks according to whether she found them useful or not.

5. Having Cindy do "research" on the old story, especially on the rules that perfectionism used to remain strong.

The Story Re-Vision Process

1. Juxtaposing the old story with the new story in terms of the differences in specifications and rules between the two, and the stories' differing usefulness for Cindy's life. This was made possible in three ways:

2. Locating evidence of the new story via identifying unique outcomes, accounts, redescriptions, and possibilities.

3. Searching for, and finding, guidelines that could serve to inform the new story.

4. Generating strategies to counteract the influences of perfectionism.

Keeping the Re-Vision Alive and Well

1. Using a reflecting team at the specification-burning ritual, to provide an appreciative and validating audience for the new story.

2. Providing Cindy with a tape of the burning ritual.

3. Inviting Cindy to attend a session as a consultant and helper to the therapist, which cast her as an expert on change.

4. Gaining her permission to use her story in this book—a story that would prove helpful to others.

5. Using therapeutic letters at various stages in the therapy to document Cindy's performance of a new story.

We should note that this is certainly not the "one and only true form" of a case following a narrative analogy. Rather, it is one story among the many that could be written. It is offered as an example, or better yet a metaphor, which we hope will aid the reader's understanding of our work.

CHAPTER 6

The Re-Vision of Therapists' Stories in Training and Supervision

Therapists are very much like their clients. They too, have old stories and other past influences that have contributed to their sense of personhood and view of the world. Just like their clients, they are influenced by fear, uncertainty, self-depreciation, and anger, although usually (but not necessarily!) to a lesser extent. And, like their clients, therapists are sensitive to interactions with others that they experience as invasive and insensitive to their stories. This seems especially accurate in reference to situations in which a therapist is "talking to herself/himself" about a really difficult case, or is receiving supervision and training from other therapists. In the same way that therapists can "be violent" with their clients by demanding that the clients accept a certain point of view, they can also be violent with themselves and with those they have been asked to supervise.

It has been our experience that supervision, especially for a beginning therapist, is one of the major influencing elements in the development of a story concerning one's professional identity. Just as in childhood, if supervision and interactions with colleagues invite a stance of shame and guilt during a person's "therapist infancy," it is likely that some type of personal story will result. Thus, we find some supervisees resorting to passive, victimized, and avoidant stories, while others depend upon angry, rebellious, and defiant accounts. Regardless of the type of personal narrative developed, however, it is all too common to find unspoken feelings of self-doubt, insecurity, and shame ("I may not be good enough") existing in relationship to a supervisional stance that invites such feelings. Perhaps one has only to remember one's own early years as a therapist, and the type of supervision received during that period, to indentify personally with this issue.

The implications of this line of thinking for therapists, therapist supervisors, and consultants have been intriguing to us. This is especially so in respect to the model of narrative therapy we have attempted to outline in this book. In this model, clients are viewed as participants in an ongoing story or drama, and a wondering stance is used by therapists to help facilitate client change. Questioning is used as a means of gathering information and of opening space for story re-visions.

Frequently, however, it has been our experience that this kind of approach is not employed in the development of new stories or solutions in response to difficulties experienced by therapists and/or supervisors. Instead, it seems that therapists are often invited to lay aside the ideas and beliefs they use in therapy when they are trying to be useful to colleagues or to themselves. This seems equally often to be accompanied by a habitual return to more lineal, static, and causative lines of reasoning. When this occurs, therapists have moved away from the subjunctive mode (the "as if" or "might be" mode) and have inadvertently fallen prey to the indicative mode (the "this is the way it is" mode). The indicative mode is primarily concerned with conformity—telling others how things are, with the intent that they will accept this story and adopt it as their own. Such an emphasis on conformity is a prevailing "grand narrative" in our society and culture, and inevitably invites shame on the part of those who are unable to comply.

A previous publication (Clifton, Doan, & Mitchell, 1990) has presented our initial ideas on self-management, supervision, and consultation, using the same narrative model that we employ with our clients. The purpose of this chapter is to expand upon that work, and to provide readers with a sufficient base for experimenting with these ideas in their own clinical settings, should they be interested in doing so. In developing these notions we have relied heavily on Gregory Bateson's (1980) concept of "double description," as well as on the work of Michael White and David Epston (White & Epston, 1989; White, 1989).

As previously pointed out, Bateson's concept of double description has become an integral part of doing family therapy from a narrative stance. He proposed that "difference which makes a difference'' is a necessary component in the problem-solving process, and that this is best generated by contrasting two or more descriptions of the same sequence of events. As stated by Bateson (1980), "it takes at least two somethings to create a difference" (p. 76).

White and Epston (White, 1988a, 1988b, 1989, 1991; Epston, 1989a; Epston & White, 1992) have extended this notion of multiple descriptions by developing an entire therapy based upon eliciting and documenting multiple descriptions from their clients. Our own work, as outlined in this book, is consistent with the idea that reality as we know it is only one interpretation among many that could have been selected. A story re-vision is literally an exercise in entertaining multiple descriptions of the sequence of events a person selects to represent his/her lived experience. This has as many implications for therapists as it does for clients, in our opinion.

In supervising therapist students and trainees over the years, we have come to believe that this process commonly involves three major areas of concern and interest. These can be summarized as the stories therapists have about their clients, about themselves, and about other therapists. In addressing these areas, we present ideas on (1) the re-vision of therapists' stories about their clients; (2) the re-vision of their stories about themselves as therapists; and (3) helping other therapists re-vision their stories about themselves. Once again, we provide an appendix of what we hope are helpful suggestions, dialogues, and questions at the end of the chapter.

THE RE-VISION OF THERAPISTS' STORIES ABOUT CLIENTS

As family therapists, we encounter a very diverse and difficult population in the course of doing our jobs, and since we are human beings as well as therapists, it is highly improbable that we will like all the clients we have occasion to meet. Some clients are just more difficult than others, although which types are experienced as difficult will vary, depending upon the therapist in question. In our own practices, as well as in the stories we have heard from our students, some clients are not only difficult; they also invite us to side with the notion that we are not very good therapists. Most counselors are familiar with this type of client, and medical-model diagnostic labels such as "borderline," "hysterical," "antisocial," and "conduct-disordered'' come to mind in reference to them. In traditional models of therapy, this type of client might also be conceptualized as ''resistant.'' Difficult cases present therapists with very strong invitations to ''know about the clients,'' as well as to begin to doubt their own effectiveness. We have not been able to understand how either of these accounts are useful for the therapeutic process. Instead, we have found it more helpful to remember to ask ourselves, and our students, questions that invite a different sort of storying of clients. The following is a representative list of such questions:

• If, instead of being viewed as stubborn or resistant, I saw this client as being stuck in a childhood story in which he/she is afraid, how would my story about the client change?

• If, instead of seeing this client as obnoxious, I saw her/him as trying to tell me something important, what might that something be?

• If my boredom with this case were telling me that I have stopped being curious, and have inadvertently bought into the notion that I know the truth about this client, how would my perceptions change? (Stewart & Parry, 1989)

• If I were more sensitive to the situation that my clients are in, and less tightly bound to a model of therapy, what might I notice that has gone unseen before?

• How am I making sense of my client's life that is different from how he/she sees it? What factors and influences might have led to his/her view that I need to understand?

• Is the gender of the client, or my gender, coloring my story about her/him in a significant way?

• What sort of story does the diagnostic label that has been applied to this case by others invite the client and me to participate in? Is the label doing most of the authoring? What evidence do I have that supports alternate descriptions of the client?

• Am I more interested in helping this person discover a story that will work for him/her, or in fulfilling some personal agenda that has to do with my own life?

Questions such as these are based on the notion that what has been commonly understood as ''pathology'' is actually a particular type of story itself, and that it, like everything else, can be viewed from various other perspectives. ''Pathological'' and ''resistant'' clients are called forth by a story that could be entitled "Following the Medical Model for Fun and Profit," and exist only in the particular set of meanings and interpretations accompanying such a narrative. In other words, each of us is contantly involved in the "performance of meaning" (White, 1988–1989), which becomes the lens through which we view our world. As long as such views end in a "period" instead of a "question mark," so to speak, no other possibilities are available to us. We hope that our work is characterized by the attempt to keep a question mark at the end of most observations we make about our clients. (See the end-of-chapter appendix for additional comments in this regard.)

THE RE-VISION OF THERAPISTS' STORIES ABOUT THEMSELVES

As previously mentioned, there are times when therapists are invited to feel overwhelmed, incompetent, and self-doubting. This is often a multifaceted process involving several elements of the therapists' lives. Frequently, this can include a separation from a story or a time in which they believed in themselves. When such a separation is combined with the influence of an authority that introduces a new set of dominant specifications to define their success as persons and as professionals, then a sense of being "outside a story of competence" can follow. We suggest that this description is often accurate of new therapists and trainees, as well as of experienced therapists who are studying under some well-known "master." In such instances, as therapists encounter dominating styles of teaching or supervision, it is quite common for them to misplace accounts about themselves in which they are competent. When this occurs, the therapists can be viewed in much the same light as clients who have been highly influenced to let others author their stories, rather than to rely on their own perceptions and experience. We have found the following questions and reminders helpful in combating such negative influences and stories about our professional roles.

• If I were looking at myself through the eyes of my clients, what would I be seeing in me that they appreciate?
• I am asking my clients to become much better at identifying ways in which they can successfully escape from a problem-satur-

ated story. Can I experiment along with them in being able to do that myself?

• Would it be OK if I consistently acknowledged my resources and strengths? Would this be part of a solution for me, or have I been trained to be "allergic" to success? If I have been so trained, what would be necessary to overcome this allergy?

• How is it that I have allowed another's experience of my work to carry more weight than my own experience? What was *my* experience of the session that this other person thinks was so bad?

• Can I be sure and remember to forget my strengths and resources every morning when I arise?

• How much of my time as a therapist do I spend trying to avoid feelings of shame and not being good enough? What standard of "therapist conformity" does this shame exist in relationship to?

HELPING OTHER THERAPISTS RE-VISION THEIR STORIES

In consulting with and supervising other therapists, we have been very interested in helping them become the types of helpers they desire to be, rather than in encouraging them to conform to some story that we hold about what they should be. We have experimented with the use of subjunctive (wondering) questions and assignments to accomplish this end. Our intent has been to expedite the process of their writing stories that have competent therapists as the central characters. The subjunctive mode allows a process of "active imagining" (Stewart & Parry, 1989), which can be used in the story re-visions. The focus of such imagining is to render distinct at least two possible stories about being a therapist. For example, this process can be used to draw distinctions between a story about a competent hero/heroine and one about an incompetent victim. Such a stance encourages therapists to view themselves as being in the process of becoming, rather than as needing to have arrived somewhere. In other words, it invites therapists to entertain the difference between being a "thing" and being part of a "process." This line of thinking fits well within the narrative analogy, in that stories are processes within which change inevitably occurs. Some of the questions previously presented can be utilized in this process, as well as those listed below.

- Who has been the major author (or authors) of your story as a therapist? Where did the initial invitations to view yourself as incompetent come from?
- If 1,000 people were to read a novel about your life as a therapist, what would they understand to have been the major influences contributing to the story line? How would they understand that these influences have invited you to think, act, and feel?
- Which do you think is most in charge of your professional life at present: a competent therapist journey, a victim role, or a rebellious adolescent script?
- Can you think of times as a therapist that you have escaped the influence of incompetence and insecurity, and instead opted to side with your strengths instead?

Over the past few years, we have been experimenting with training therapists from the stance outlined above. This has been done in a training group of 8–10 members supervised by one of us. Within this context, we have been able to present various role plays, assignments, and forms of feedback designed to invite the trainees to re-vision their therapist texts. We have found this to be a very powerful experience for all those involved. The various ideas that have been implemented are as follows:

1. The trainees are asked to write accounts of the characters they are now playing in their therapist stories. Within these accounts they are to consider aspects of their stories they would like to change or alter, as well as those they would like to remain the same. They are also asked to include what they feel are the major outside influences that have been instrumental in authoring their stories.

2. In role-play exercises, the trainees "do therapy" with each other in which a "therapist" asks questions that call forth the story a "client" is playing in her/his professional life. The "therapist" then experiments with documenting the story by writing it, and presents it to the "client" for comments and corrections. We have found this to be a particularly useful exercise for both parties involved, as it includes practicing the model and applying the model to oneself simultaneously. It should be noted that this exercise is limited to information about the "client's" life as a therapist, rather than aspects of her/his more personal existence; the person being interviewed is instructed to share only the information that seems comfortable for

her/him. The intent of this exercise does *not* include being invasive or intruding on the trainees' personal lives.

3. The trainees are asked to use active imagining to conceptualize the steps they could take that would cooperate with a process of re-vision concerning their stories about themselves as therapists. Some possible steps are presented to them as examples: (a) pretending to be a different character and role-playing a session from that position; (b) playing the therapist they would like to be and videotaping themselves for later review; and (c) watching videotapes of themselves in which they attend *only* to those aspects of themselves that they would like to keep and promote.

4. Two reflecting teams are used, with one team providing feedback to the client(s), and the other providing feedback to the therapist in a postsession setting. Reflecting teams can also be used in a role-play format in which the primary purpose of the team is to provide feedback and wonderings for the therapist. The teams are instructed to concentrate on the aspects of the therapist's behavior that are most like the ones he/she has indicated a desire to keep. Again, Chapter 4 has provided a more complete discussion of the reflecting team's purpose and function.

5. In occasional group meetings, the trainees share stories about their experiences as therapists. These include how they came to be involved in this type of work, the changes in what it means to them to be therapists that have occurred over time, and the areas in which they feel they have made significant improvement.

6. We suggest that when the trainees are doing live sessions with reflecting teams observing, they make at least three "mistakes" during the session. We have been amazed that our trainees tell us this is one of the most helpful aspects of the training! Similarly, we always try to convey the message that each person works uniquely, and that therapy sessions conducted by one person will vary from those conducted by others. Even identical premises "look different" when filtered through a particular therapist's personality. Some narrative therapists work from a very "laid-back" orientation, while others operate "on the edge of their seats" (Epston, 1989b).

CONCLUDING COMMENT

The story or narrative that we call "Supervision" can take many different forms. We believe that in traditional contexts, it has often taken on an interpretation in which the supervisor is the expert and the trainee is somehow deficit. This version of supervision is highly analogous to the traditional relationship between the therapist and client, in which the therapist is seen as "knowing" and the client is seen as "not knowing" and in need of "treatment." Thus, in dealing with stories or interpretations about clients, about ourselves as therapists, and about others as therapists, we have been interested in a re-vision of the story titled "Supervision" that stresses the same sort of stance we seek to take with our clients. In this version, the supervisor is seen as an editor, a catalyst—as one who helps "call forth" the type of therapist the trainee wishes to be, rather than as one who defines the type of therapist she/he should be. This story is still in process for us; it is as yet incomplete. New lines and chapters are being written regularly, as we learn from our interactions with others in the process of supervision and training. We hope that it will always remain so.

APPENDIX: THERAPEUTIC EXAMPLES

The Re-Vision of Therapists' Stories about Clients

Sample Case Notes

In reference to keeping a "question mark" at the end of most observations we make about our clients, we have found it helpful to ask ourselves the following: "Would we be comfortable in letting our clients see the case notes we have made concerning them? If we did so, would they find them helpful, expanding, and thought-provoking, or would they feel judged and misunderstood?" The result of asking such questions has changed the format of the notes we take—and enabled us to feel very comfortable sharing these notes with the clients at the end of the session if they so desire. The following case note examples serve to illustrate the difference between notes taken with "periods" and those that stress "question marks."

Notes Taken from a "Knowing" Stance ("Period" Notes)

This couple's relationship is obviously dominated by gender stereotypes. The male is very dominant and patriarchal in his attitudes, while the female is passive and must resort to covert, manipulative strategies to gain power in the relationship.

Notes Taken from a "Curious" Stance ("Question Mark" Notes)

I find myself wondering to what extent this couple has been influenced by cultural notions concerning traditional male and female roles. Were their families of origin organized according to stereotypical gender specifications? How comfortable is this couple with such roles? Would one or both partners desire change in this area, or are such roles satisfactory for them?

In the second set of notes, the therapist has made an effort to suspend judgment and knowing in favor of curiosity and wonderment. If such notes are shared with clients, the invitation is for them to tell their story, rather than for the therapist to assume that he/she already knows what it is. Such notes can become an extension of the therapeutic conversation, and can be sent home with the clients as a form of intervention. They can also be utilized by the therapist/editor as a basis for subsequent sessions.

Supervision Dialogue Examples

In this section we present some actual dialogues that took place in the context of a therapist training group. There were six therapists/trainees in attendance, and the purpose of the session was to discuss and re-vision stories about the clients they were currently experiencing as the most difficult. The reader may notice that the re-vision of stories about clients often overlaps with the re-vision of stories that therapists are telling themselves in response to such clients.

Supervision Dialogue 1

The therapist in the first instance was a female in the 35–45 age range. The client she was most concerned about was a 17-year-old male. The therapist was somewhat distraught that after three sessions the client still showed no signs of trusting her; moreover the parents of the adolescent did not want to be involved in the therapy, and showed no signs of being willing to change anything in the home environment. The family had a long history of physical abuse, and the client had been the recipient of much of the violence. After an investigation by a state agency, the case was dismissed. This was also of great concern to the therapist. The supervision comments and questions were offered by five different group members, but are incorporated below under the general heading of "Supervisor."

SUPERVISOR: So up to this point in time, what has it meant to you that you have not been able to establish a relationship with this client?

THERAPIST: It has meant that I don't have enough experience . . . that I'm doing something wrong.

SUPERVISOR: And how much has the relationship with this client gotten you to believe that this is the case?

THERAPIST: Uhmm . . . probably about 75% of the time.

SUPERVISOR: So instead of considering that the issue may be this particular client's past, and the unstable and violent relationships which have been part of it, you have been telling yourself that the issue is primarily one of your inability.

THERAPIST: Well, not totally. I am usually very good at establishing relationships with my clients. I think that most of them trust me.

SUPERVISOR: So how have you managed to hold onto this knowledge? I mean, you could be totally telling yourself that if you were worth a damn, three sessions is enough . . . how have you managed to fight this off to the extent that you have?

THERAPIST (*laughing*): I don't know, I really don't. I guess I've postponed judging it entirely . . . that I've decided to wait and see.

SUPERVISOR: It sounds like you are siding with the notion that around 75% of the issue is your fault, however. How would you view it differently if it was 50–50?

THERAPIST: I'd be less hard on myself . . . I wouldn't expect so much.

SUPERVISOR: How would it be different if the story line read that it would even be dangerous for this client to trust too quickly . . . that it might not even be good for him?

THERAPIST: Instead of seeing him as difficult, and myself as defective, I would be more inclined to let him be the guide on the pace of our relationship.

SUPERVISOR: So knowing what you do about yourself—that you have good relationships with most of your clients—what information would this give you about yourself?

THERAPIST: That I tend to vacillate between feeling overwhelmed and . . . I know that's not good.

SUPERVISOR: Vacillate between being overwhelmed and what? You didn't tell us what the other was.

THERAPIST: And not telling myself scary stories.

SUPERVISOR: So which invites you to experience this case as difficult the most: the feeling that the client doesn't trust you, or that Mom and Dad aren't going to help and they're not going to change?

THERAPIST: Mom and Dad, that's more than the other.

SUPERVISOR: So it's not only the relationship you are having with the client; it's also that nothing you can do will make any difference at home.

THERAPIST: Yes, that's a big part of it.

SUPERVISOR: Let's say that is an accurate story. What kind of things could you tell yourself so that you could be the most helpful to your client?

THERAPIST: My role is not to fix the family in this case . . . because I may not even be allowed in the door.

SUPERVISOR: So what would your role be?

THERAPIST: I guess it would be to help this young man cope until he is grown . . . to provide him with a relationship which is not like those he has at home, and to invite him to see that he doesn't have to be that way either.

SUPERVISOR: What would it mean if you did that?

THERAPIST: In this case, it would mean that I could be very happy with what I'd done.

Supervision Dialogue 2

The therapist in the second example was also a female. The client was a young adult mother who was very depressed as a result of a tragic and oppressive past, which had left her feeling almost totally incompetent. The therapist was hopeful of being able to help this woman re-vision her story, but had been told by her supervisor that the case was too difficult and should be referred to a psychiatric agency.

THERAPIST: I don't know how to start with this client. There are so many things going on . . . she's depressed, and she feels very inadequate as a parent. She describes her relationship with her husband as feeling very much like the one she was in while she was growing up.

SUPERVISOR: So what is overwhelming you is that there are too many things to address and you don't know where to start?

THERAPIST: Yes.

SUPERVISOR: What if there were only one thing to address? Would that be helpful?

THERAPIST: Yes, I'd start with that one . . . I might feel less overwhelmed. I think maybe also that part of the problem is that I don't want to reject this person by sending her off to some other agency, but my agency thinks I should. She resists that idea—she seems to want to work with me. She has kept all of her appointments with me, which is different than what she has done in the past.

SUPERVISOR: Sounds like your story is different from your agency's.

THERAPIST: Yeah. Not that I don't see that she's had a very sad life and that it might be a difficult story to change, but there are some things about her that give me hope for her.

SUPERVISOR: I'm feeling confused . . . I don't know if anyone else is or not. My understanding was that this case was brought up because it was a very difficult client. What I've heard so far is that in spite of a very bad past, and in spite of her agency, the therapist is still hopeful about this client and wants to work with her. Is anyone else confused about this? What is making this client difficult? Is it the way you feel about her, the way she feels about herself, or the way that others feel about her?

THERAPIST: It's been partly all of that . . . it's been pressure to deal with the case in ways that aren't comfortable to me.

SUPERVISOR: What kind of story have you been telling yourself about you as a therapist which invites you to think you could help this woman?

THERAPIST: Well . . . I think that the hope that I see in her is the hope that she sees in me. Does that make sense? She's been through a series of clinicians . . .

SUPERVISOR: And are you the first one who has been hopeful?

THERAPIST: I don't know, but she's here and she's saying things like "Can you help me?"

SUPERVISOR: It sounds like—and I'm guessing—that she has been not only through a series of therapists, but also through a series of people who have totally discounted her voice. That she's never had anyone to validate her story. And that even now while her voice is saying that she wants to work with you, others are trying to tell her that she is wrong . . . that she should be sent somewhere else. You may be the first person to have really heard her.

THERAPIST: That's probably pretty accurate, from what she tells me.

SUPERVISOR: So how important would it be to you as a female to model for her things like confidence, trusting your own voice . . . showing her a strong female voice?

THERAPIST: That would be very important to me.

SUPERVISOR: I can't help but wonder how important it would be not only for her voice to be considered valid, but for yours to be as well. Are your perceptions of her and this case valid? Or can someone steal those from you?

THERAPIST: That's something I've struggled with a long time.

SUPERVISOR: But in this case you have found your own voice . . . you are in touch with what type of work you'd like to do with her. What is your perception of your opinion when compared to those of others?

THERAPIST: I'm feeling more comfortable in here. This process is giving validity to my opinions whereas I haven't experienced that where I work.

SUPERVISOR: Gosh, you must understand exactly how she feels!

THERAPIST: Yeah, I guess I do. Maybe I need to get stronger in believing in myself too . . . and not let what others think influence me so much.

SUPERVISOR: As you are able to do that, will this case seem easier or harder?

THERAPIST (*smiling*): Easier. I would be more at peace.

The Re-Vision of Therapists' Stories about Themselves

The following example was excerpted from a dialogue that one of us had with a trainee. It demonstrates the interviewing techniques that we like to practice while supervising other therapists.

SUPERVISOR: John, I don't know why you're here today, I only know that you requested a meeting with me and that you are concerned about something.

THERAPIST: Well, let me just tell you straight off, I'm concerned about this new practicum I've been offered. I want to do well, but I'm not certain that I can.

SUPERVISOR: So if you labeled what you're feeling, would it be fear, anxiety . . . what would you call it?

THERAPIST: It would be fear . . . it's really affecting me these days.

SUPERVISOR: So, it's fear. It sounds like it's even been trying to take away some of the joy of the accomplishment of getting selected for this practicum.

THERAPIST: Yes, it is. When it is in control, I don't even want to accept the position.

SUPERVISOR: So it gets so strong as to suggest that you not even do the practicum?

THERAPIST: Yeah, it kind of gets me to doubting myself—worrying that I will end up looking dumb in front of other people.

SUPERVISOR: It sounds sort of like the clients that we see. Fear can be just as tricky with us as it is with them. It can take all the joy away.

THERAPIST: It has sure been doing that.

SUPERVISOR: How much of the time has fear been able to steal the joy of accomplishment away?

THERAPIST: Well, when I really think about it . . . oh, probably about 30% of the time.

SUPERVISOR: Really? The other 70% interests me. What is the difference between the two? What is going on during the 70% that is not during the 30%?

THERAPIST: The 30% seems unreasonable. I mean, how likely is it to really happen? The 70%—well, I feel comfortable with my abilities. I feel confident about myself.

SUPERVISOR: During that 70%, are you more in touch with the person who successfully completed a master's degree and got offered this practicum over lots of other applicants?

THERAPIST: Yeah, I guess so . . . I hadn't thought of it that way.

SUPERVISOR: But during the 30% that fear is in charge, it somehow manages to get you to lose touch with the person who did all that.

THERAPIST: Yes, I guess it does. During that time, it's like I'm this shy guy from a small town, a country boy. Who do I think I am, trying to impress people who really know how to do therapy?

SUPERVISOR: If I remember right, you had a conversation with a nationally known therapist who got to watch you work. Do you remember that conversation?

THERAPIST (*smiling*): Yeah, I sure do.

SUPERVISOR: What would she say about this practicum opportunity?

THERAPIST: She would offer some encouragement . . . some type of reassurance. She was real positive about my potential.

SUPERVISOR: I wonder what she is seeing in you that you lose sight of during this 30% of the time.

THERAPIST: I guess she appreciates my ideas . . . thinks that they are worth hearing.

SUPERVISOR: If you were to began to appreciate what she appreciates, what difference would it make in thinking about this practicum?

THERAPIST: I don't know. Maybe if I just tried to be comfortable with my ideas and skills . . . just presented them for what they are . . . maybe that's the difference it would make.

SUPERVISOR: It sounds like that would be more in line with this story of competence you have about yourself most of the time.

THERAPIST: Yes, it would.

SUPERVISOR: I'm surprised that you have managed to hold on to this story of competence 70% of the time, in spite of fear's best efforts. Were you aware you were doing this?

THERAPIST: No, fear had managed to convince me that I was feeling fearful most of the time.

SUPERVISOR: Uhmm . . . that's interesting, isn't it? That fear can really be the lesser portion but feel like the larger.

THERAPIST: Yeah, it is.

SUPERVISOR: So now that you are more aware of its actual influence on you, what do you think? Will the 30% win out, or do you want to side with the 70%?

Helping Other Therapists Re-Vision Their Stories

As outlined in the chapter text, we have been experimenting with various ideas within the context of a therapist training group. Here, we present various examples of the results of this process.

*2. Role-Play Interviews Exploring
a Trainee's Professional Identity*

The following is an actual letter written to one of our trainees as a result of being interviewed by one of her colleagues. Such letters are then discussed by the two people involved, and needed changes or additions are made.

Dear Jane Doe,

I enjoyed visiting with you last Wednesday to discuss your ideas about your identity as a counselor. It sounds as if self-doubt, and to a lesser extent confusion, are at times quite successful at invading your life and your perceptions of your ability as a counselor. In fact, they seem to have cleverly teamed up to invite you to even question your decision about being in this area of work at all! When under their influences, which seems to occur fairly regularly (like the "steady beating of a bass drum"), you tend to side with a story of uncertainty and questionable competence regarding your potential to become a good therapist.

You are not entirely at their mercy, however. You shared that along with the bass drum, the sound of an irregularly beating snare drum can also be heard. The snare drum allows you to escape self-doubt and encourages you to side with a story about yourself as a competent counselor. I'm curious about how you are able to listen to the snare drum over the pounding confusion of the bass? I wonder how it would be for you if the stories associated with the bass and the snare could change places—if the snare drum were to become what you hear most of the time? I'm also curious about how much of the time the sound of the snare drum is there, but it gets overlooked because of the power of the bass. Is it possible that the snare is beating much more often than you realize?

I hope this is a reasonable account of our conversation. If I have left something out, or misunderstood anything, please correct it for me. I hope that we will have the opportunity to visit about this topic in the next month or so. I will look forward to being updated on your progress! [Thanks to Susan Lasuzzo for this letter.]

4. The Use of a Reflecting Team That Reflects to the Therapist

Reflecting teams can be just as powerfully used in the opening of space for story re-visions in therapists' lives as they can for clients. The following is an example of such reflections. They will not be as pertinent as they might be, since the reader will not have heard the therapy session that preceded them. However, we hope they will serve to illustrate the type of information that can be shared in such a process.

TEAM MEMBER 1: I know that before the session that Jill said she was very nervous . . . that this was her first time to do a solo session in front of the group. However, she didn't appear nervous to me as I observed her. I wonder if she is aware of how well she controlled nervousness, or would she think that she hadn't?

TEAM MEMBER 2: Yes, I noticed that as well. The part of the session which really impressed me was when after about 20 minutes of the session had transpired, she returned to something the client had said in the first minute! This really interested me . . . nervousness sure didn't seem to affect her memory. I wonder how she was able to focus so well in spite of it?

TEAM MEMBER 1: Yes, and also the fact that the client didn't present with what we had been led to believe that she would. It was something entirely unexpected. Jill seemed able to go right with this and to explore her story anyway. I found myself wondering if I would have been able to adjust that quickly . . . and what it means about her that she did?

TEAM MEMBER 3: In our interactions with Jill, we have learned that one of her goals is to do narrative therapy in such a way that it fits with her personality—with who she is—rather than try and copy any of our styles. I wonder if she feels she was able to do that during this session? From my perspective, I thought that she did. She was very gentle and kind during the session, and took great care not to steal the client's voice away from her. It is my understanding that these are things that are important to her as a counselor. I am curious as to how she feels that she did in this regard. How would she rate herself?

TEAM MEMBER 4: I was very impressed that even during periods when she was experiencing the session as being difficult, she remained calm. I thought it was wonderful that at one point she very calmly asked the team to phone in any ideas that they might have! I would hope that I would be able to be so spontaneous and creative in using the team. I find myself wondering whether Jill is telling herself that asking the team to call is proof of failure, or if she is in touch with how creatively she used our presence? I guess I'm wondering what sort of story she's telling herself about this.

TEAM MEMBER 2: Yes, I liked that as well. Instead of us having to wonder whether we should call her, she let us know. As it turned out, we had some ideas that were worth exploring. Her openness in asking us for input during the session added to the therapy, in my opinion. In fact, I've been wondering if we shouldn't start operating that way more of the time—you know, let the therapist ask for the team to call, rather than us just doing so when we have an idea.

5. Occasional Group Meetings in Which Trainees Share Their Therapist Stories

We have found that the sharing of stories about trainees' experiences as therapists is most powerfully accomplished by bringing in a "consultant" therapist—one who has not been a part of the group, but who is intensely interested in hearing the stories of the members. In our case, since we reside in very different settings (Doan in Edmond, Oklahoma, and Parry in Calgary, Alberta), we are able to use each other in that manner. Parry has been kind enough to attend the training group that Doan is part of in Oklahoma, and to elicit stories from the various group members. We were both amazed at the response he received from his simple yet salient opening question: "I am interested in your stories about how it came to be that you are part of this group, and how this group has contributed to your journey as a family therapist. Would you be interested in sharing these stories with me?" This invited the members to make their stories more real by relating them to an audience of interested listeners. It also served to document the journeys they had been making by inviting them to reflect on where they had been, as opposed to where they were currently. Many of them noted afterward that they had not realized how much improvement they had made until they told their stories, that in the telling, the awareness materialized. We highly recommend this process as a powerful component in the process of story re-visioning.

References

Adler, A. (1956). *The individual psychology of Alfred Alder* (H. L. Ansbacher & R. E. Ansbacher, Eds. and Trans.). New York: Harper & Row.

Alexander, R. (1989). Evolution of the human psyche. In P. Mellars & C. Stringer (Eds.), *The human revolution*. Princeton, NJ: Princeton University Press.

Amundson, J., & Stewart, K. (1993). Temptations of power and certainty. *Journal of Marital and Family Therapy, 19*(2), 111–123.

Andersen, T. (1987). The reflecting team: Dialogue and meta-dialogue in clinical work. *Family Process, 26,* 415–428.

Anderson, H., & Goolishian, H. (1990, November 16). *New directions in systemic family therapy: A language systems approach.* Workshop presented in Tulsa, OK.

Auden, W. H. (1966) In memory of Sigmund Freud. In W. H. Auden, *Collected shorter poems, 1927–1957.* London: Faber & Faber. (Original work published 1939)

Bateson, G. (1972). *Steps to an ecology of mind.* New York: Ballantine Books.

Bateson, G. (1978). The birth of matrix or double bind and epistemology. In M. M. Berger (Ed.) *Beyond the double bind: Communication and family systems, theories and techniques with schizophrenics.* New York: Brunner/Mazel.

Bateson, G. (1979). *Mind and nature: A necessary unity.* New York: Bantam Books.

Berg, I. K. (1992, April 30). *Solution focused brief therapy.* Workshop sponsored by High Pointe Treatment Center, Edmond, OK.

Bergman, J. (1985). *Fishing for barracuda: Pragmatics of brief systemic therapy.* New York: Norton.

Bly, R. (1990) *Iron John: A book about men.* Reading, MA: Addison-Wesley.

Borges, J. L. (1964). Tlon, Uqbar, Orbis Tertius. In D. A. Yates & J. E. Irby (Eds.), *Labryrinths: Selected stories and other writings.* New York: New Directions. (Original work published 1961)

Brown, N. O. (1966). *Love's body.* New York: Random House.

Bruner, J. (1986). *Actual minds, possible worlds.* Cambridge, MA: Harvard University Press.

Bruner, J. (1990). *Acts of meaning.* Cambridge, MA: Harvard University Press.

Campbell, J., & Abadie, M. J. (1984). *The mythic image.* Princeton, NJ: Princeton University Press.

Clifton, D., Doan, R., & Mitchell, D. (1990). The reauthoring of therapists' stories: Taking doses of our own medicine. *Journal of Strategic and Systemic Therapies, 9,* 61–66.

Coale, H. W. (1992). The constructivist emphasis on language: A critical conversation. *Journal of Strategic and Systemic Therapies, 11*(1), 12–26.

de Shazer, S. (1982). *Patterns of brief family therapy.* New York: Guilford Press.

de Shazer, S. (1985). *Keys to solutions in brief therapy.* New York: Norton.

de Shazer, S. (1988). *Clues: Investigating solutions in brief therapy.* New York: Norton.

de Shazer, S., Berg, I., Lipchik, E., Nunnally, E., Molnar, A., Gingerich, W., & Weiner-Davis, M. (1986). Brief therapy: Focused solution development. *Family Process, 25,* 207–221.

Doan, R. (1991). Investigating specifications for personhood: Escaping the influence of role rigidity. *The Calgary Participator, 1*(2), 18–20.

Doan, R., & Clifton, D. (1990, Winter). The rules of problem lifestyles: Making externalizations more real. *Dulwich Centre Newsletter,* pp. 18–21.

Eliade, M. (1958). *Rites and symbols of initiation: The mysteries of birth and rebirth.* New York: Harper & Row.

Epston, D. (1986). Night watching: An approach to night fears. *Dulwich Centre Review,* pp. 28–39.

Epston, D. (1989a). *Collected papers.* Adelaide, Australia: Dulwich Centre Publications.

Epston, D. (1989b, February 10). *The narrative model: Therapy on the edge of your seat.* Workshop sponsored by Family and Children's Services, Tulsa, OK.

Epston, D., & White, M. (1992). *Experience, contradiction, narrative, and imagination.* Adelaide, Australia: Dulwich Centre Publications.

Fisch, R., Weakland, J. H., & Segal, L. (1982). *The tactics of change: Doing therapy briefly.* San Francisco: Jossey-Bass.

Foucault, M. (1980). *Power/knowledge: Selected interviews and other writings 1972–1977* (C. Gordon, Ed.; C. Gordon, L. Marshall, J. Mephan, & K. Soper, Trans.). New York: Pantheon Books.

Gadamer, H.-G. (1976). *Philosophical hermeneutics* (D. E. Linge, Ed. and Trans.). Berkeley: University of California Press.

Garcia Marquez, G. (1970). *One hundred years of solitude* (G. Rabassa, Trans.). New York: Harper & Row.

Glantz, K., & Pearce, J. K. (1989). *Exiles from Eden: Psychotherapy from an evolutionary perspective.* New York: Norton.

Goolishian, H., & Anderson, H. (1988). Human systems as linguistic systems: Preliminary and evolving ideas about the implications for clinical theory. *Family Process, 27,* 371–393.

Guralnik, D. B. (Ed.), (1982). *Webster's new world dictionary.* New York: Simon & Schuster.

Haley, J. (1973). *Uncommon therapy*. New York: Norton.

Hoffman, L. (1989, September 16). *My 25 years as a family therapist*. Workshop sponsored by High Pointe Treatment Center, Oklahoma City, OK.

Hoffman, L. (1990). Constructing realities: An art of lenses. *Family Process*, *29*, 1–12.

Howard, G. (1989). *A tale of two stories: Excursions into a narrative approach to psychology*. Notre Dame, IN: Academic Publications.

Howard, G. (1991). Cultural tales: A narrative approach to thinking, cross-cultural psychology, and psychotherapy. *American Psychologist, 46*(3), 187–197.

Howard, G. (1992, October 30–31). *Stories, stories everywhere, and not a truth to think*. Workshop sponsored by the University of Central Oklahoma, Edmond, OK.

Humphrey, N. (1976). The social function of intellect. In P. P. G. Bateson & R. A. Hinde (Eds.), *Growing points in ethology*. New York: Cambridge University Press.

Imber-Black, E. (1988). Idiosyncratic life cycle transitions and therapeutic rituals. In E. Carter & M. McGoldrick (Eds.), *The family life cycle: A framework for family therapy*. New York: Gardner Press.

Irigaray, L. (1974). *Speculum of the other woman* (G. C. Gill, Trans.). Ithaca, NY: Cornell University Press.

Irigarary, L. (1986). The fecundity of the caress. In R. A. Cohen (Ed.), *Face to face with Levinas*. Albany: State University of New York Press.

Irigaray, L. (1991). *The Irigaray reader* (M. Whitford, Ed.). Cambridge, MA: Blackwell.

Jameson, F. (1981). *The political unconscious: Narrative as a socially symbolic act*. Ithaca, NY: Cornell University Press.

Jameson, F. (1991). *Postmodernism, or the cultural logic of late capitalism*. Durham, NC: Duke University Press.

Jenkins, A. (1990). *Invitations to responsibility: The therapeutic engagement of men who are violent and abusive*. Adelaine, Australia: Dulwich Centre Publications.

Keen, S. (1991). *Fire in the belly: On being a man*. New York: Bantam Books.

Keen, S., & Fox, A. V. (1989). *Your mythic journey*. Los Angeles: Tarcher Books.

Kinman, C. (1993, April). *Conflicting discourses: Therapeutic conversations with youth involved with substance misuse*. Paper presented at Narrative Ideas and Therapeutic Practice Conference sponsored by Yaletown Family Therapy, Vancouver, British Columbia.

Kinman, C. (1994). "If you were a problem": Consulting those who know about the tactics of a problem. *Journal of Child and Youth Care, 9*(2).

Levinas, E. (1991). *The Levinas reader* (S. Hand, Ed.). Cambridge, MA: Blackwell.

Levinas, E., & Kearney, R. (1986). Dialogue with Emmanuel Levinas. In R. A. Cohen (Ed.), *Face to face with Levinas*. Albany: State University of New York Press. (Original work published 1974)

Lipchik, E. (1988, Winter). Interviewing with a constructive ear. *Dulwich Centre Review*, pp. 3–7.

Lipchik, E., & de Shazer, S. (1986). The purposeful interview. *Journal of Strategic and Systemic Therapies, 5,* 88–99.

Lowe, R. (1991, Autumn). Postmodern themes and therapeutic practices: Notes toward the definition of "Family Therapy: Part 2." *Dulwich Centre Newsletter,* pp. 41–52.

Lyotard, J.-F. (1984). *The postmodern condition: A report on knowledge* (G. Bennington & B. Massumi, Trans.). Minneapolis: University of Minnesota Press.

Mair, M. (1988). Psychology as story telling. *International Journal of Construct Psychology, 1,* 125–137.

MacIntyre, A. (1981). *After virtue: A study in moral theory.* Notre Dame, IN: University of Notre Dame Press.

Maturana, H. (1978). The biology of language: The epistemology of reality. In G. Miller & E. Lenneberg (Eds.), *Psychology and biology of language and thought.* New York: Academic Press.

McHale, B. (1992). *Constructing postmodernism.* London: Routledge.

Menses, G., & Durrant, M. (1986). The application of the principles of cybernetic therapy to the residential treatment of irresponsible adolescents and their families. *Journal of Strategic and Systemic Therapies, 5,* 3–15.

Miller, D., & Lax, W. D. (1988). Interrupting deadly struggles: A reflecting team model for working with couples. *Journal of Strategic and Systemic Therapies, 11,* 1–11.

Nabokov, V. (1962). *Pale fire.* New York: G. P. Putnam Sons.

Nichols, M. & Schwartz, R. (1991). *Family therapy: Concepts and methods.* Boston: Allyn and Bacon.

Nietzsche, F. (1968). *Twilight of the idols* (R. J. Hollingdale, Trans.). Harmondsworth, Middlesex, England: Penguin Books. (Original work published 1889)

Nussbaum, P. (1988). Narrative emotion: Beckett's genealogy of love. In S. Hauerwas & L. G. Jones (Eds.), *Why narrative? Readings in narrative theology.* Grand Rapids, MI: William B. Eerdmans.

Parry, A. (1990). Story-connecting: What therapy is all about. *The Calgary Practitioner, 1*(1), 12–14.

Parry, A. (1991a). A universe of stories. *Family Process, 30,* 37–54.

Parry, A. (1991b). Shared stories: The tie that binds. *The Calgary Participator, 1*(3), 17–21.

Patrick, J. (1991). Meaning and purpose in medicine: The physician in a disenchanted world. *Humane Medicine, 7*(3), 195–201.

Polkinghorne, D. E. (1988). *Narrative knowing and the human sciences.* Albany: State University of New York Press.

Pynchon, T. (1973). *Gravity's rainbow.* New York: Viking Press.

Ricoeur, P. (1984). *Time and narrative* (Vol. 1). Chicago: University of Chicago Press.

Ricoeur, P. (1991a). Life: A story in search of a narrative. In M. J. Valdés (Ed.), *A Ricoeur reader: Reflection and imagination.* Toronto: University of Toronto Press. (Original work published 1987)

Ricoeur, P. (1991b). Poetry and possibility. In M. J. Valdés (Ed.), *A Ricoeur reader: Reflection and imagination.* Toronto: University of Toronto Press. (Original work published 1982)

Rogers, C. (1957). The necessary and sufficient conditions of therapeutic personality change. *Journal of Consulting Psychology, 21,* 95–103.

Rorty, R. (1989). *Contingency, irony and solidarity.* New York: Cambridge University Press.

Rorty, R. (1991). *Objectivity, relativism and truth: Philosophical papers* (Vol. 1). New York: Cambridge University Press.

Rushdie, S. (1981). *Midnight's children.* London: Jonathan Cape.

Selvini Palazzoli, M., Boscolo, G., Cecchin, G., & Prata, G. (1980). Hypothesizing–circularity–neutrality: Three guidelines for the conductor of family interviews. *Family Process, 19,* 3–12.

Sheinberg, M. (1992, September). *Families, violence and incest: Treatment of battering and incest from a gender perspective.* Lecture–workshop sponsored by the Alberta Association of Marriage and Family Therapy, Edmonton.

Stewart, B., & Nordrick, B. (1990). The L. D. lifestyle: From reification to liberation. *Family Therapy Case Studies, 5,* 61–73.

Stewart, B., & Parry, A. (1989, April 7–8). *Psychosystemic therapy: Two steps forward, one step right.* Workshop sponsored by the Edmond Counseling and Training Center, Edmond, OK.

Stone, E. (1988). *Black sheep and kissing cousins: How our family stories shape us.* New York: Penguin Books.

Tappan, M. B., & Brown, L. M. (1989). Stories told and lesson learned: Toward a narrative approach to moral development and moral education. *Harvard Educational Review, 59*(2), 182–205.

Tomm, K. (1989). Externalizing the problem and internalizing personal agency. *Journal of Strategic and Systemic Therapies, 8,* 54–59.

Tomm, K. (1990). *Questions to an "internalized other" that open new clinical possibilities.* Paper presented at S. K. Littmann Psychiatric Research Day, Foothills Hospital, Calgary, Alberta.

Tomm, K. (1991). Beginnings of a HIPs and PIPs approach to psychiatric assessment. *The Calgary Participator, 1*(2), 21–24.

Turner, V. (1969). *The ritual process.* Ithaca, NY: Cornell University Press.

vanGennep, A. (1960) *The rites of passage.* Chicago: University of Chicago Press.

White, M. (1983). Anorexia nervosa: A trans-generational perspective. *Family Process, 22*(3), 255–273.

White, M. (1984). Pseudo-encopresis: From avalanche to victory, from vicious to virtuous cycles. *Family Systems Medicine, 2,* 150–160.

White, M. (1986). Negative explanation, restraint, and double description: A template for family therapy. *Family Process, 25,* 169–184.

White, M. (1988a, Autumn). Assumptions and therapy. *Dulwich Centre Newsletter,* pp. 5–7.

White, M. (1988b, Winter). The process of questioning: A therapy of literary merit? *Dulwich Centre Newsletter,* pp. 3–20.

White, M. (1988–1989, Summer). The externalization of the problem and the re-authoring of lives and relationships. *Dulwich Centre Newsletter,* pp. 3–20.

White, M. (1989, May 11). *Reauthoring of selves and relationships.* Workshop sponsored by Family and Children's Services, Tulsa, OK.

White, M. (1991, Autumn). Deconstruction and therapy. *Dulwich Centre Newsletter,* pp. 21–40.

White, M., & Epston, D. (1989). *Literate means to therapeutic ends.* Adelaide, Australia: Dulwich Centre Publications.

Whitman, W. (1950). Song of myself. In J. E. Miller, Jr. (Ed.), *Walt Whitman: Complete poetry and selected prose.* Boston: Houghton Mifflin. (Original work published 1855)

Zimmerman, J. (1992, September 16). *An overview of narrative therapy.* Workshop sponsored by the VA Hospital, Oklahoma City, OK.

Zimmerman, J., & Dickerson, V. (in press). Narrative therapy and the work of Michael White. In M. Elkaim (Ed.), *Thérapies similes: Les approches principales.* Paris: Editions du Seuil.

Zukav, G. (1989). *The seat of the soul.* New York: Simon & Schuster.

Index

Abandonment, fear of, 132–133
Abusive experiences, and survival
  stories, 38–39, 41
Adolescents, conflictual problems with
  parents, 75–80, 161
Anger, 95–96
  in hurtful situations, 88–90, 133–134,
  155
Audience for new stories, 158–167
  and clients speaking to groups, 172,
  185
  in interviews with client, 163–166, 176
  in interviews with significant others,
  162–163, 175–176
  in letters to significant others,
  161–162, 173–175
  reflecting team as, 62–63, 166–167,
  177–179
  therapeutic examples of, 173–185
Avoidant behavior, protective function
  of, 134–135

Biblical stories, 2, 5, 23
Blaming of victims, 53
Brain development, and adaptation to
  social environment, 33–35

Case history as literary genre, 8
Childhood
  and children as characters in family
  stories, 37
  protection and preparation in, 35,
  38–39, 72–75, 115–116
  reality testing in, 35–36
  rites of passage in, 42
  as source of later difficulties, 33
  survival stories in, 38–39, 133
  unspeakable events as unstoried
  reactions in, 39

Christian stories, tyranny of, 37–38
Cindy's case
  background of, 48–49
  and client as consultant for others, 173
  deconstruction process in, 185–186
  development of rules for new story in,
  58–59, 93–94
  externalization of problems in, 54
  identification of dominant themes in,
  51
  re-vision process in, 186
  reflecting team used in, 62–63, 167,
  177–179
  research on power strategies in old
  stories, 55–56
  specifications of personhood in, 57–58
  survival of new story in, 166
  unique redescriptions in, 106–107
Cognitive questions, 13
Collision of stories, 68
  conflict management in, 75–80,
  116–117
  individual stories in, 48
Comparison of old and new stories,
  questions used in, 175–176
Conflict
  between adolescents and parents,
  75–80, 161
  management in collision of stories,
  75–80, 116–117
Connectedness of all stories, 28, 48,
  162–163
  and sharing of connections that have
  been secret, 69, 114
Consciousness, landscapes of, 108
Consensual belief in one single truth,
  loss of, 9, 16, 20, 28
Conspiratorial points of view, prevalence
  of, 9–10
Constraints
  in dominant story lines, 17

212

in old stories, 40–42
    specifications of personhood in,
        56–58, 92
    and unseen power strategies, 54–56,
        90–92
Consultants, clients as, 172–173
Conversation as enacted narrative, 3
Cybernetics, 15, 24, 35, 128, 137, 142
Cyberpunk writers, 10, 20

Deconstruction
    connectedness of stories in, 28
    and emotional beliefs about reality, 37
    in externalization of old story, 53
    linked to re-vision, 45
    process in, 42–43
Demarginalization of groups, 10, 20, 23
Depression as symptom from old story
        line, 128, 150–151
Dominant stories
    challenges to, 5–6
    as expanded focus in therapy, 126
    gender in, 130
    reinterpretation of, 50
    as themes in new stories, 49–51, 84–86
    tyranny of, 17–18, 37–38
Double descriptions of same events,
        188–189

Emotions as narrative constructs, 36–38
Epistemological questions, 13, 15, 21, 23
Ethics, postmodern, 30–33
Evolutionary psychology, 33–34, 38
Externalization of old stories or
        problems, 5, 17, 41–42, 52–54
    therapeutic examples of, 86–90

Family
    analysis of story types in, 70–72,
        114–115
    as crossroads, 26, 30, 190
    different stories and different lan-
        guages in, 26, 29–30
    only one story in, 72
    protective and preparative parenting
        in, 72–75, 115–116
    rituals in, 30
    shared stories in, 29–30
    in "talking-stick" session, 69–70, 114
    as system, 16, 21
Family therapy
    definition of, 47–48
    early developments in, 14–16
    postmodern challenges to, 18–22
    and science of interpretation, 22–26
    recent innovations in, 17–18

stories used in, 5–6
    tasks of narrative therapists in, 27–30
Fear, 95–96
    of abandonment and rejection, 132–133
Feminism, 21, 50–51, 154
Fight and flight responses in survival
        stories, 133
Freud as first narrative therapist, 7–8, 13

Gaps in stories, from forgotten ex-
        periences, 8
Gender
    in dominant stories, 130
    language differences in, 154
    sensitive stance maintained by ther-
        apists, 129–130, 152–154
    stereotypical specifications for, 56,
        195–196
Grand narratives
    to legitimize paradigmatic systems, 4
    loss of authority in, 9–11
    and development of personal
        narratives, 24–25
    patriarchy in, 20, 53
    presented as normal ideas, 47
    tyranny of, 5, 25, 28–29
Group meetings for therapists, 194,
        204–205

Hermeneutics, 22–23, 44
Hidden texts in stories, 39–41, 128
    tracked by reflecting team, 132–135,
        155
Hurtful situations, anger in, 88–90,
        133–134, 155
Hyperspace, 11, 12

Intentionality, 3, 6, 80–83, 117
Internalization of others, 5, 7–8
    and sense of victimhood, 10
Interpretations
    alternate, in telling of multiple stories,
        59–60, 96–97
    compassionate misreading in, 29
    different possibilities in, 44
    and discipline of hermeneutics, 22–23
    in perception of reality, 22
    reinterpretation of dominant themes,
        50
    by therapists, 47
Interviews
    with client, 163–166, 176
    role-play, for trainee therapists,
        202–203
    with significant others, 162–163,
        175–176

Jumping ahead in new stories, effects of, 168–169

Labeling of clients, 52–53, 65, 87, 129, 138–139, 189–191
Landscapes of action and of consciousness, 107–108
Language
and formation of agreements, 16, 19
gender differences in, 154
narrative, 4
paradigmatic, 4
Legitimacy of personal stories, 26–27
Letters
to consolidate new story roles, 167–168, 179–181
to significant others, 161–162, 173–175
therapeutic, 18, 127
Liberating stories, 5–6

Many selves and many stories for each person, 18
liberation of, 27–29
Meaning constructions of clients, exploration of, 128–129, 152
Meaningfulness of stories affecting credibility, 2
Metanarrative. *See* Grand narratives
Miracle questions, responses to, 67, 108–111
Moral dimension of stories, 2–3
Motivations. *See* Intentionality
Multiple versions of same events, 188–189
alternate interpretations in, 59–60, 96–97
reflecting team as source of, 135–136

Narrative traditions, credibility of, 1–4
Neurobiologic factors in behavior, 33–35
New stories. *See also* Re-vision
audience for. *See* Audience for new stories
development of rules for, 58–59, 93–96
effects of jumping ahead in, 168–169
letters to consolidate roles in, 167–168, 179–181
maintenance of, 157–186

Old stories or problems
constraints in. *See* Constraints
externalization of, 5, 17, 41–42, 52–54, 86–90

as only one story, 64–65
rules for, compared to new stories, 58–59, 93–96
scouting reports on strategies in, 55–56, 90–92
Ontological questions, 13, 15, 21, 23
Optionality, and choice between stories, 71–72
Others
clients in therapy sessions for, 172–173, 185
demarginalization of, 10, 20, 23
internalization of, 5, 7–8
responsibility for, as ethical challenge, 30–33
seen as less human, 34
sharing of stories with, 32–33

Paradigmatic cognition, 2, 4–5
Patriarchy, 20, 32, 53
Periods opposed to question marks, in punctuation as metaphor, 60–61, 138, 191, 195
Perspectives, limitations of, 24
Play as practice for survival, 35, 38–39
Postcognitive questions, 14
Power
lack of, from conspiracies, 9–10
and operation of giant systems, 25
pervasiveness of, 17
in unexamined stories, 71
and unseen strategies in problem stories, 54–56, 90–92
Preparative parenting, 35, 38–39, 72–75, 115–116
Pretended roles in new stories, 63–64, 99
Problems, separation of persons from, 17, 52
Protective parenting, 35, 38–39, 72–75, 115–116
Psychotherapy
assumptions and therapeutic aims in, 12–14
scientific language in, 4
Punctuation as metaphor, periods opposed to question marks in, 60–61, 138, 191, 195

Reality
perceptions of, interpretations in, 22
testing in childhood, 35–36
Reciprocal invitations, 76–77, 87–88, 161
Reflecting teams, 62–63, 130–136, 155–156, 194, 203–204
as audience for new story, 166–167, 179–181

open discussions with therapists, 136
open-ended stories of, 136
reflections written for clients, 136
as source of multiple stories, 135–136
to track hidden texts, 132–135, 155
Rejection, fear of, 132–133
Resistant clients, 124, 142–143
labeling of, 65, 138, 139, 190
Re-vision
alternate interpretations in, 59–60,
96–97
basis for, 43
and clients as experts on story
changes, 170–173, 182–185
continuation of, 157–186. *See also* Audience for new stories
documenting progress in, 64–67,
99–108
in externalization of old story, 53
importance of, 45–47
linked to deconstruction, 45
new pretended roles in, 63–64, 99
and responses to miracle questions, 67,
108–111
rituals in, 61–63, 97–99
therapist as editor in, 118–130
of therapists' stories, 187–195
stories about clients, 189–191,
195–200
stories about themselves, 191–192,
200–202
therapeutic examples of, 195–205
unique outcomes in, 66–67, 100–102
Rituals
in families, 30
in rites of passage, 42
in story re-vision, 61–63, 97–99
Rules
established by families, 35, 54
in fear and anger lifestyles, 95–96
for new stories, development of,
58–59, 93–96

Sacred stories, 4–7, 9
Scouting reports on power strategies in
old stories, 55–56, 90–92
Self
defined by external sources, 56
esteem of, 9
gratification in consumer society, 14,
25, 31
as motivating force, 13
Shared stories
in families, 29–30
in "talking-stick" sessions, 69–70,
114
related to individual stories, 48

Social learning, rules of interaction in,
35, 54
Societal consensus of truth, lack of, 9,
16, 20, 28
Solution-focused therapy, 18
Specifications of personhood
explorations of, 56–58, 92
long-standing definitions in, 65
separation from, rituals in, 61–63,
97–99
Strengths of clients, listening for, 66,
125, 143–144
Supervision of therapists, re-vision of
stories in, 187–195
therapeutic examples of, 195–205
Supporting roles in stories of others
children as characters in family stories,
37
collision of stories in, management of,
67–69, 111–114
and demarginalization of groups, 10,
20, 23
symptoms attached to, 128, 149–151
therapists as editors of, 120–121
Survival stories, 38–39
anger as hurt in, 88–90, 133–134
applied to current situations, 52
avoidant behavior in, 134–135
deconstruction of, 42
fight or flight response in, 133
hidden texts in, 40
old stories affecting, 28
Systemic family therapy, 16

"Talking-stick" sessions for sharing of
stories, 69–70, 114
Therapists
asking "what would it mean" questions, 128–129, 152
attentive listening by, 50–51, 66, 122
"coin-flip" interventions of, 111
compassion of, 123, 140
curiosity of, 122–123, 138–139, 146
expanded focus of, 125–126, 144–146
as experts, 8
focus on symptoms from old story
line, 128, 149–151
gender-sensitive stance of, 129–130,
152–154
group meetings for, 194, 204–205
helping other therapists in re-vision of
stories, 192–194, 202–205
information gathered by, 123–124,
140–141
intentions of, examination of, 81
interpretations by, 47

Index

Therapists (*continued*)
  labeling of clients, 65, 87, 129
  neutrality of, 121–122, 136–138
  permission ''not to know,'' 126–127,
    139, 146
  in reflecting teams, 130–136
  and resistance of clients, 65, 124,
    142–143
  re-vision of therapists' stories, 187–205
  as re-visionary editors, 118–130
  staying behind new stories, 168–169,
    181–182
  tasks in family therapy, 27–30
  transparency in work with clients, 132,
    136
  watching for clients' strengths, 66,
    125, 143–144
  working harder than clients, 127,
    146–149
Time as factor in narratives, 3
Timing of rituals, 98
Trust, and childhood development,
  38–39
Truth
  lack of societal consensus on, 9, 16,
    20, 28
  and perceptions of reality, 22
  universal, pursuit of, 2, 10–12, 31
Tyrannizing stories, 5–6, 17–18, 37–38

Unconscious, 8, 13, 36
Unique outcomes
  encouragement of, 17–18
  found in lost stories, 27–28
  in re-vision, 66–67, 100–102
Unique possibilities, therapeutic
  examples of, 104–106
Unique redescriptions, therapeutic
  examples of, 102–104
Unspeakable events. *See* Hidden texts in
  stories

Victimhood
  blaming of victims in, 53
  conspiratorial themes in, 9–10
  powerlessness in narratives of, 26
Videotapes of clients, 171–172, 182–185

Wake-up calls, 42, 44, 61, 149
Women, subordination of, 32
Writers
  and art in closed fields, 15
  conspiratorial themes of, 10
  postmodern views of, 5, 19